Healthy Diet for Healthy Pregnancy

The Ultimate Cookbook for Moms to Be

BY: SOPHIA FREEMAN

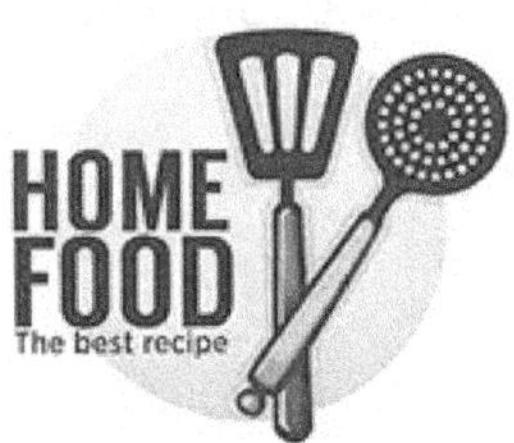

Liability

This publication is meant as an informational tool. The individual purchaser accepts all liability if damages occur because of following the directions or guidelines set out in this publication. The Author bears no responsibility for reparations caused by the misuse or misinterpretation of the content.

Copyright

The content of this publication is solely for entertainment purposes and is meant to be purchased by one individual. Permission is not given to any individual who copies, sells or distributes parts or the whole of this publication unless it is explicitly given by the Author in writing.

Table of Contents

Introduction

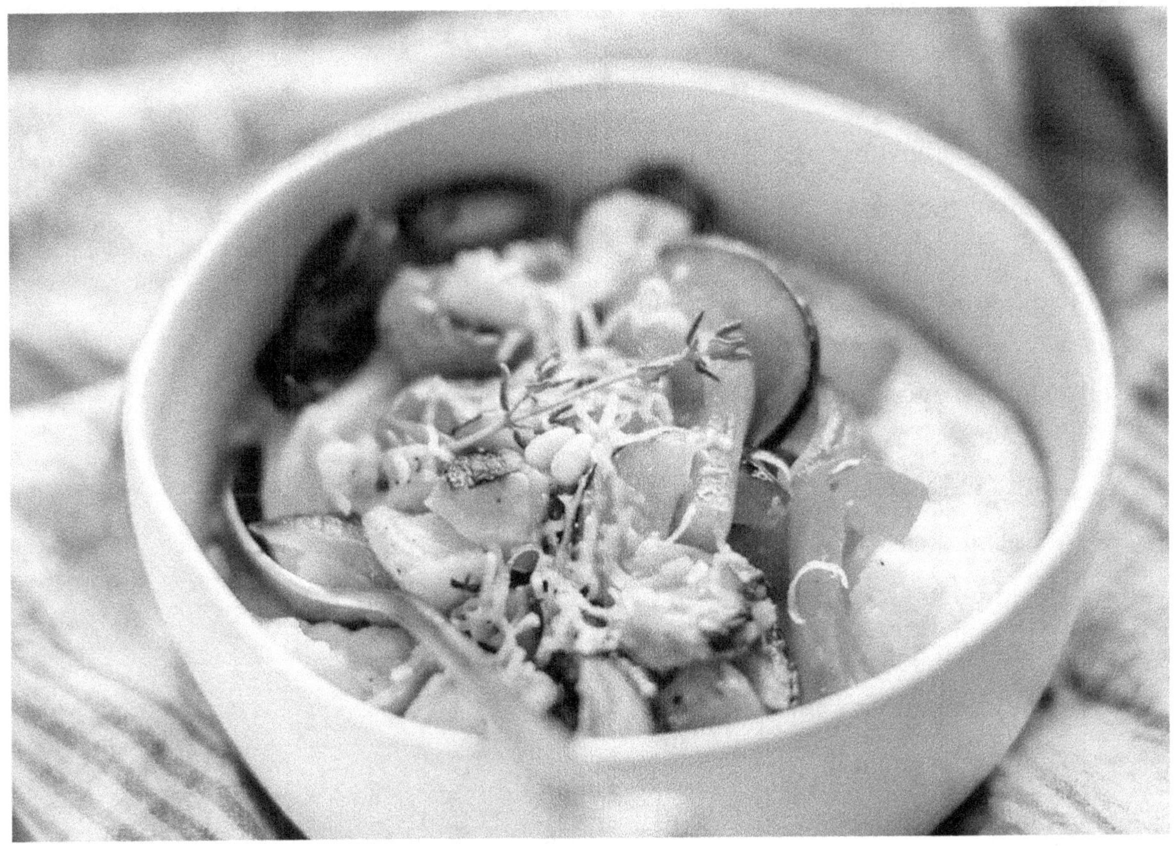

Eating for two?

When you're pregnant, there are many things that you have to think about—baby supplies and equipment, birthing and delivery, easing morning sickness, and so on.

But that's not all.

Besides, you need to make sure that you are getting the right nutrients because you are not only eating for yourself, but also nourishing the baby inside your womb.

Proper diet has been known to have many benefits for both the mother and the baby.

For the mother, a healthy diet can help improve unpleasant pregnancy symptoms such as morning sickness, mood swings and fatigue. This can also greatly help during labor and delivery.

For the baby, a healthy diet can lower the risk of birth defects and ensure proper development of the brain.

Now the question is: what is a well-balanced diet?

A well-balanced diet for pregnancy includes sufficient intake of the following:

- Fruits and vegetables
- Whole grains
- Healthy fats
- Foods rich in protein
- Foods high in vitamin C
- Foods with calcium
- Foods high in iron and folic acid

Moreover, it's also important to know that there are certain types of food that pregnancy women should avoid.

Here are some of those:

- Cold cuts
- Processed meat
- Rare or undercooked meat
- Undercooked eggs (e.g. runny yolks)
- Fish high in mercury (e.g. swordfish, mackerel)
- Sushi
- Raw fish and shellfish
- Smoked seafood
- Coffee
- Alcohol

Eating anything that's raw or not cooked properly may expose you to bacteria such as Listeria that has been proven dangerous for the fetus, increasing the risk of stillbirth, miscarriage and preterm labor.

This book provides you with recipes that are not only highly nutritious but also won't endanger the safety of your little one.

It's time to get started.

Squash Lasagna

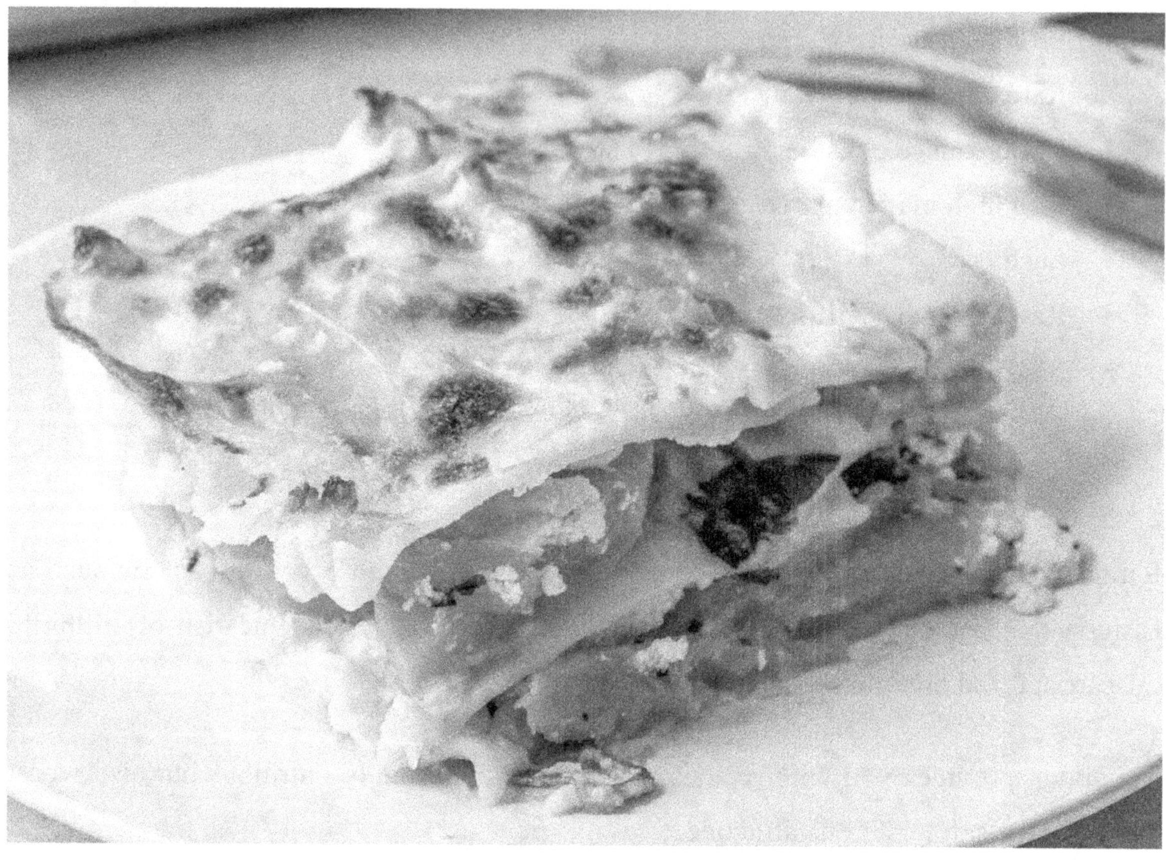

Do you love lasagna? For sure, you're going to have fun preparing this unique lasagna version that trades lasagna noodles with butternut squash slices. The dish is packed with vegetables and creamy cheese sauce.

Serving Size: 8

Preparation Cooking Time: 2 hours

Ingredients:

- 3 cups nonfat milk, divided
- ½ cup all-purpose flour
- 1 cup Parmesan cheese, grated
- 3 tablespoons low-fat cream cheese
- ⅛ teaspoon ground nutmeg
- Salt and pepper to taste
- ½ cup ricotta
- 20 oz. spinach, chopped
- 2 tablespoons olive oil
- 1 onion, chopped
- 8 oz. white mushrooms, sliced
- 2 cloves garlic, crushed and minced
- 1 teaspoon dried marjoram
- ½ cup dry white wine
- Cooking spray
- 2 lb. butternut squash, sliced into thin rounds
- ½ cup Italian cheese, shredded

Instructions:

1. Pour 2 ½ cups milk into a pan over medium heat.

2. Simmer until it starts to bubble.

3. In your bowl, combine the remaining milk with the flour.

4. Stir into the steaming milk.

5. Cook for 1 minute.

6. Remove from the stove.

7. Stir in the cream cheese, Parmesan cheese, nutmeg, salt and pepper. Set aside.

8. In another bowl, combine the ricotta and spinach. Set aside.

9. Pour the oil into a pan over medium high heat.

10. Cook the onion and mushrooms for 5 minutes.

11. Add the garlic.

12. Season with the salt, pepper and marjoram.

13. Cook for 1 minute while stirring.

14. Pour in the wine and reduce heat.

15. Simmer for 2 minutes.

16. Remove from the stove.

17. Preheat your oven to 400 degrees F.

18. Spray your baking pan with oil.

19. Spread ½ cup cheese sauce on the bottom of the pan.

20. Arrange the squash slices on top.

21. Top with the spinach mixture and then the mushroom mixture.

22. Repeat the layers until all ingredients have been used.

23. Top with the Italian cheese.

24. Bake in the oven for 20 minutes.

25. Lastly, let stand for 10 minutes before slicing and serving.

Nutrients per Serving:

- *Calories 288*
- *Fat 11.9 g*
- *Saturated fat 5.1 g*
- *Carbohydrates 30.6 g*
- *Fiber 4.8 g*
- *Protein 15.4 g*
- *Cholesterol 27 mg*
- *Sugars 9 g*
- *Sodium 446 mg*
- *Potassium 908 mg*

Cauliflower Buns

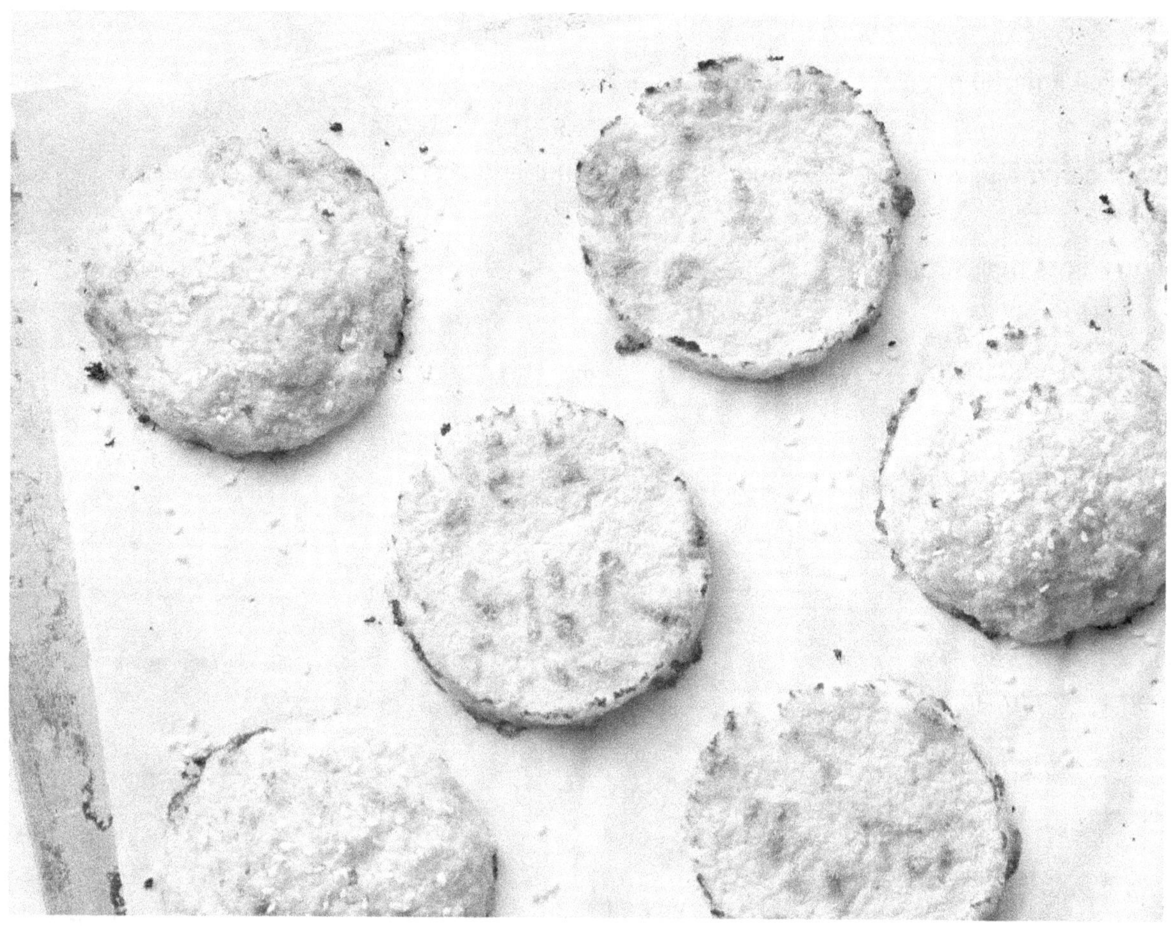

If you need to tone down your carb intake, here's a good alternative to the usual buns that you use for your burgers or sandwiches—buns made with cauliflower rice, cheese and eggs.

Serving Size: 4

Preparation Cooking Time: 45 minutes

Ingredients:

- 5 cups cauliflower florets
- 1 cup cheddar cheese, shredded
- 1 egg, beaten
- 1 teaspoon sesame seeds

Instructions:

1. Preheat your oven to 425 degrees F.

2. Line your baking pan with parchment paper.

3. Next, add the cauliflower to your food processor.

4. Pulse until finely chopped.

5. Then, microwave on high for 3 to 4 minutes.

6. Let cool.

7. Squeeze with paper towels to get rid of excess moisture.

8. Transfer to another bowl.

9. Stir in the egg and cheese.

10. Create round shapes with the mixture and place on a baking pan.

11. Bake for 25 minutes.

12. Sprinkle the buns with the sesame seeds.

Nutrients per Serving:

- *Calories 170*
- *Fat 11.4 g*
- *Saturated fat 5.9 g*
- *Carbohydrates 7.8 g*
- *Fiber 2.8 g*
- *Protein 10.7 g*
- *Cholesterol 74 mg*
- *Sugars 3 g*
- *Sodium 242 mg*
- *Potassium 442 mg*

Big Burger

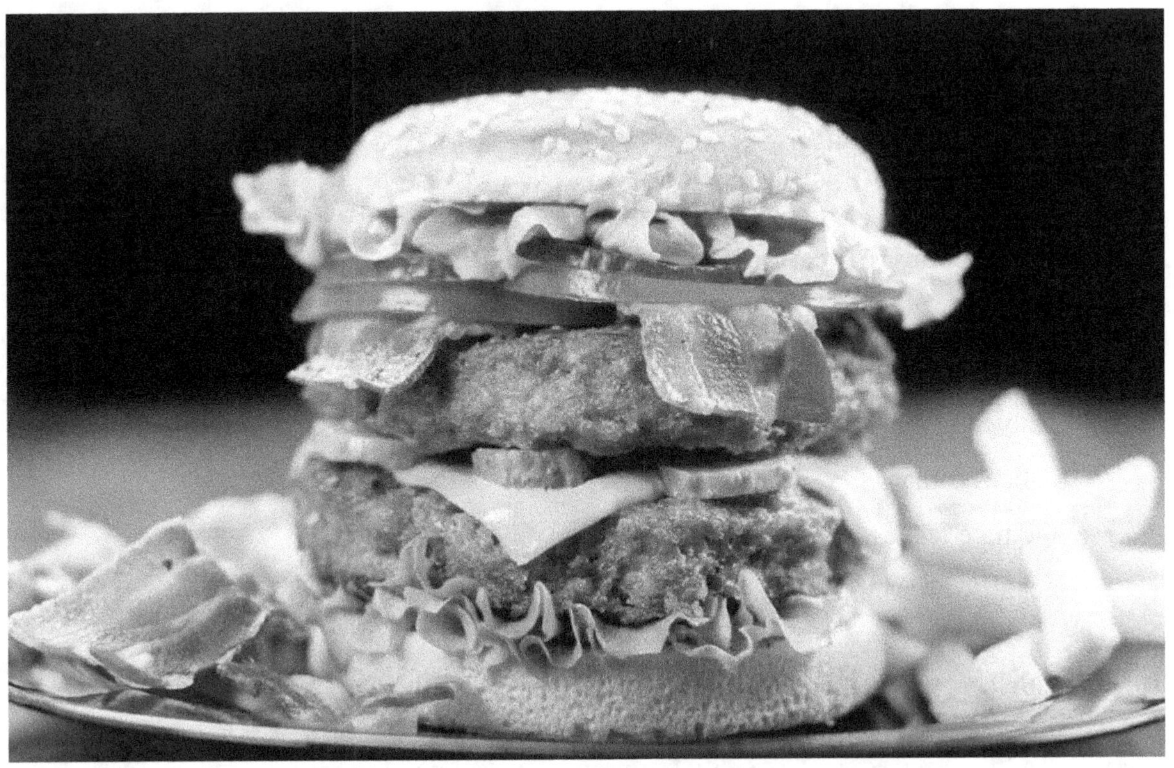

Enjoy this scrumptious burger without worrying about your carb intake. This recipe makes use of cauliflower buns that are even more delicious than the usual burger buns.

Serving Size: 4

Preparation Cooking Time: 30 minutes

Ingredients:

- 1 tablespoon vegetable oil
- 1 onion, chopped
- 2 tablespoons ketchup, divided
- 1 lb. lean ground beef
- Pepper to taste
- 2 tablespoons Worcestershire sauce
- 1 teaspoon white vinegar
- 2 teaspoons dill pickle relish
- 2 tablespoons light mayonnaise
- 4 slices tomato
- 4 lettuce leaves
- 4 cauliflower buns

Instructions:

1. In a pan over medium heat, combine the oil, onion and half of ketchup.

2. Cook for 5 minutes, stirring frequently. Transfer to a bowl.

3. Add the beef, pepper and Worcestershire sauce.

4. Mix well and form thick patties.

5. In another bowl, mix the remaining ketchup with the vinegar, pickle relish and mayonnaise. Set aside.

6. Pour the remaining oil into a pan over medium heat.

7. Cook the burgers for 7 to 8 minutes per side.

8. Assemble the burgers on the cauliflower buns with the lettuce, tomato slices and ketchup mixture.

Nutrients per Serving:

- *Calories 511*
- *Fat 31.9 g*
- *Saturated fat 11.1 g*
- *Carbohydrates 14.4 g*
- *Fiber 3.4 g*
- *Protein 42 g*
- *Cholesterol 164 mg*
- *Sugars 7 g*
- *Sodium 588 mg*
- *Potassium 983 mg*

Salmon Cucumber Salad

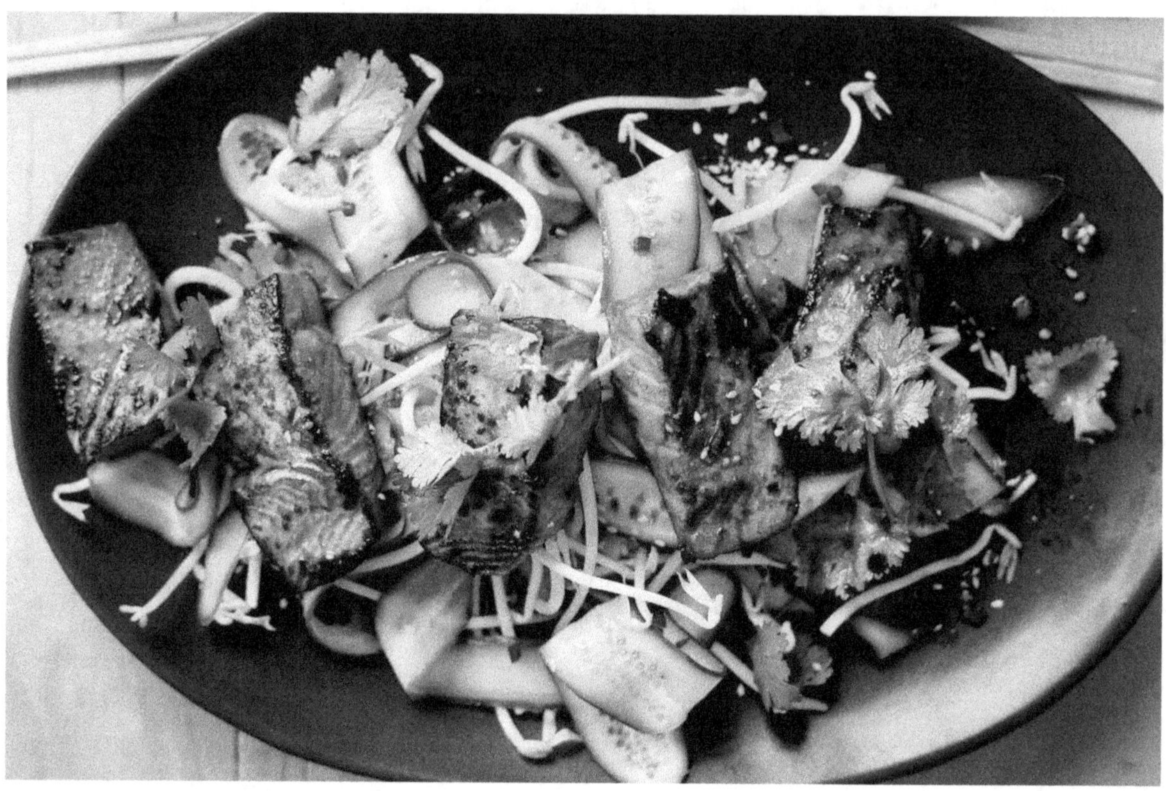

Here's a delicious grilled salmon recipe that is not only easy to prepare but also requires a few ingredients.

Serving Size: 4

Preparation Cooking Time: 20 minutes

Ingredients:

- 4 salmon fillets
- 2 tablespoons olive oil, divided
- Salt and pepper to taste
- ½ cup cucumber, sliced
- 2 tablespoons shallot, minced
- 2 tablespoons cilantro, chopped
- ¼ teaspoon curry powder
- 2 tablespoons freshly squeezed lemon juice
- ½ cup low-fat yogurt

Instructions:

1. Preheat your grill.

2. Next, brush the fish with half of the olive oil.

3. Season both sides with the salt and pepper.

4. Preheat your grill.

5. Then, grill the salmon for 4 minutes per side.

6. In a bowl, mix the cucumber, shallot and cilantro.

7. In another bowl, blend the curry powder, lemon juice and yogurt.

8. Add the cucumber mixture to the curry mixture.

9. Mix well.

10. Serve the fish with the cucumber salad.

Nutrients per Serving:

- *Calories 258*
- *Fat 12.7 g*
- *Saturated fat 2.6 g*
- *Carbohydrates 4.2 g*
- *Fiber 0.3 g*
- *Protein 30.2 g*
- *Cholesterol 68 mg*
- *Sugars 3 g*
- *Sodium 383 mg*
- *Potassium 650 mg*

Salmon with Creamy Spinach

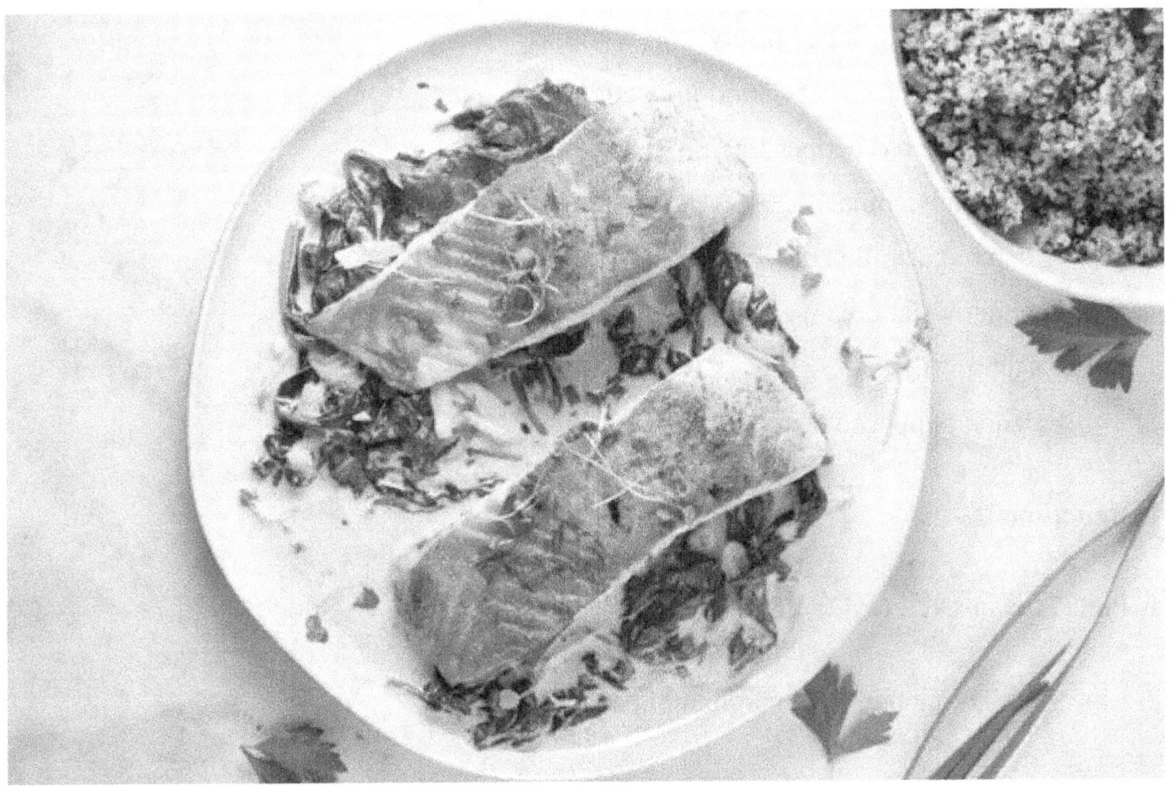

Stuff your salmon with creamy spinach not only to enhance the flavors but also to add more nutrients to your meal. The dish comes together in only 30 minutes.

Serving Size: 6

Preparation Cooking Time: 30 minutes

Ingredients:

- 1 ½ tablespoons olive oil
- ½ cup shallots, sliced thinly
- 5 cloves garlic, crushed and minced
- ¼ teaspoon red pepper flakes
- 5 cups baby spinach
- ½ cup mozzarella cheese, shredded
- ¼ cup low-fat cream cheese
- 6 salmon fillets
- Salt and pepper to taste

Instructions:

1. Preheat your oven to 425 degrees F.

2. Line your baking pan with parchment paper.

3. Pour the oil into a pan over medium heat.

4. Cook the shallots and garlic for 2 minutes.

5. Next, add the red pepper flakes and cook for 30 seconds.

6. Stir in the spinach and cook for 3 minutes.

7. Remove from the stove.

8. Stir in the cream cheese and mozzarella.

9. Remove from heat.

10. Let sit for 10 minutes.

11. Then, make a shallow cut in the middle of the fish.

12. Sprinkle with the salt and pepper.

13. Place the salmon in the baking pan.

14. Fill the cuts with the spinach mixture.

15. Bake the salmon in the oven for 10 minutes.

Nutrients per Serving:

- *Calories 312*
- *Fat 13.6 g*
- *Saturated fat 4.3 g*
- *Carbohydrates 6.5 g*
- *Fiber 1.3 g*
- *Protein 38.8 g*
- *Cholesterol 93 mg*
- *Sugars 1 g*
- *Sodium 426 mg*
- *Potassium 736 mg*

Polenta with Roasted Veggies

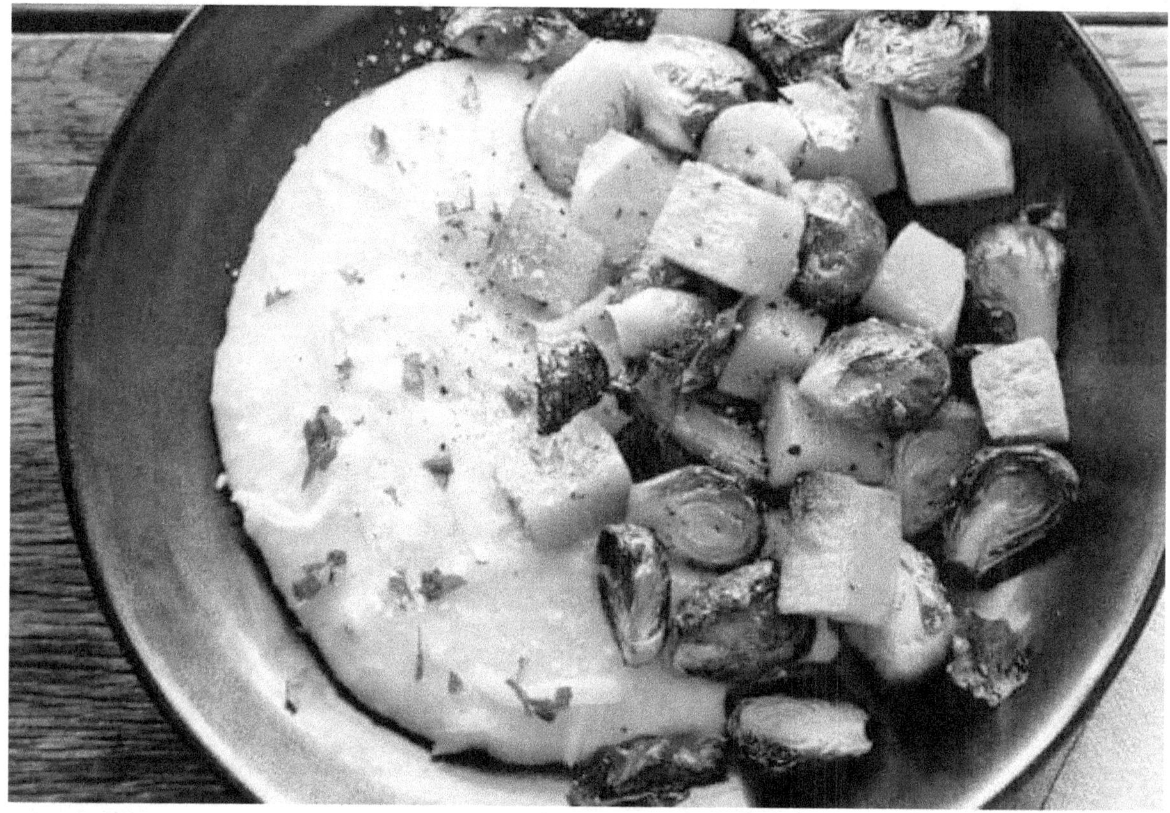

Top polenta with fried egg and serve with grilled vegetables (whatever you have in your kitchen) to create this healthy and filling meal you will enjoy.

Serving Size: 4

Preparation Cooking Time: 30 minutes

Ingredients:

- 6 shallots, sliced
- 3 tablespoons olive oil, divided
- 6 oz. mushrooms, sliced in half
- 1 lb. asparagus, sliced
- 3 tablespoons balsamic vinegar
- Salt and pepper to taste
- 1 tablespoon fresh thyme, chopped
- 2 cups chicken stock (unsalted)
- 2 cups whole milk
- ¾ cup instant polenta
- ½ cup Parmesan cheese, grated
- 4 eggs, fried (yolk fully cooked)

Instructions:

1. Preheat your oven to 425 degrees F.

2. Cover your baking pan with foil.

3. Add the shallots to the pan.

4. Toss the shallots in 1 tablespoon oil.

5. Roast for 12 minutes.

6. Next, add the mushrooms and asparagus to the pan.

7. Stir in the vinegar and 1 tablespoon oil.

8. Season with the salt, pepper and thyme.

9. Roast for 8 minutes.

10. Then, in a pan over medium high heat, cook the stock and milk.

11. Bring to a boil.

12. Stir in the polenta.

13. Reduce heat and simmer for 5 minutes.

14. Remove from heat.

15. Stir in the Parmesan cheese.

16. Serve the polenta with the fried eggs and roasted vegetables.

Nutrients per Serving:

- *Calories 453*
- *Fat 22.2 g*
- *Saturated fat 6.9 g*
- *Carbohydrates 44.2 g*
- *Fiber 4.7 g*
- *Protein 20 g*
- *Cholesterol 207 mg*
- *Sugars 11 g*
- *Sodium 674 mg*
- *Potassium 775 mg*

Taco Pizza

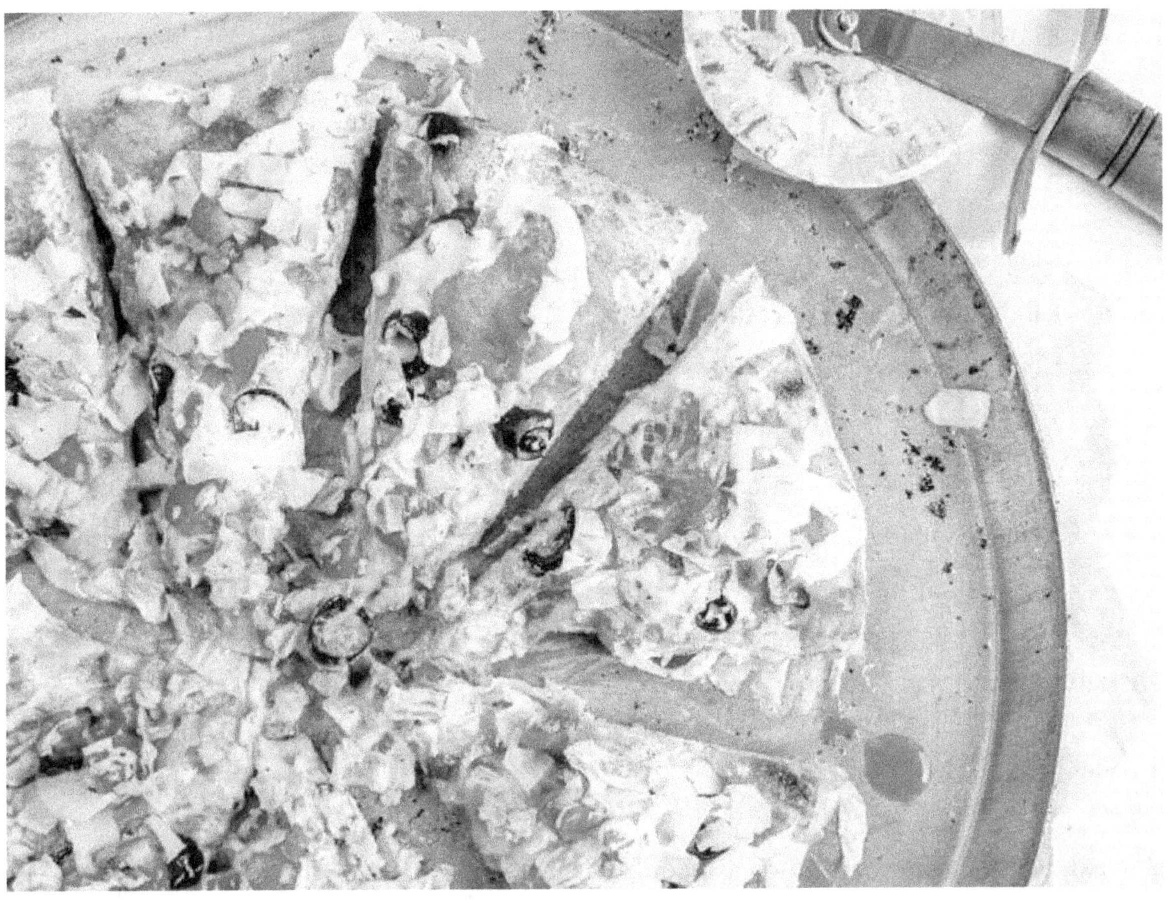

Grill this pizza topped with taco favorites like salsa and beans in a wood-fried oven for the ultimate dish that you won't get enough of.

Serving Size: 5

Preparation Cooking Time: 30 minutes

Ingredients:

- 1 lb. lean ground beef
- 15 oz. pinto beans, rinsed and drained
- Salt to taste
- 1 ½ teaspoons ground cumin
- 1 ½ teaspoons chili powder
- 1 cup salsa, divided
- 1 lb. whole-wheat pizza dough
- 1 cup Mexican cheese
- 2 tablespoons freshly squeezed lime juice
- ¼ cup sour cream
- 2 cups Romaine lettuce, shredded
- Fresh cilantro, chopped

Instructions:

1. Preheat your grill.

2. Next, add the beef to a pan over medium heat.

3. Cook for 5 minutes.

4. Stir in the beans.

5. Season with the salt, cumin and chili powder.

6. Remove from the stove.

7. Stir in half of the salsa.

8. Transfer to a bowl.

9. Spread the dough on your kitchen table.

10. Grill the dough for 2 minutes.

11. Then, spread the beef mixture on top of the crust.

12. Top with the cheese.

13. Grill for 2 minutes.

14. Combine the lime juice and sour cream.

15. Sprinkle the chopped lettuce on top along with the sour cream mixture.

16. Garnish with the fresh cilantro leaves.

Nutrients per Serving:

- *Calories 511*
- *Fat 22.4 g*
- *Saturated fat 8.4 g*
- *Carbohydrates 48.4 g*
- *Fiber 4.9 g*
- *Protein 32.9 g*
- *Cholesterol 86 mg*
- *Sugars 5 g*
- *Sodium 728 mg*
- *Potassium 548 mg*

Mushroom Spinach Quiche

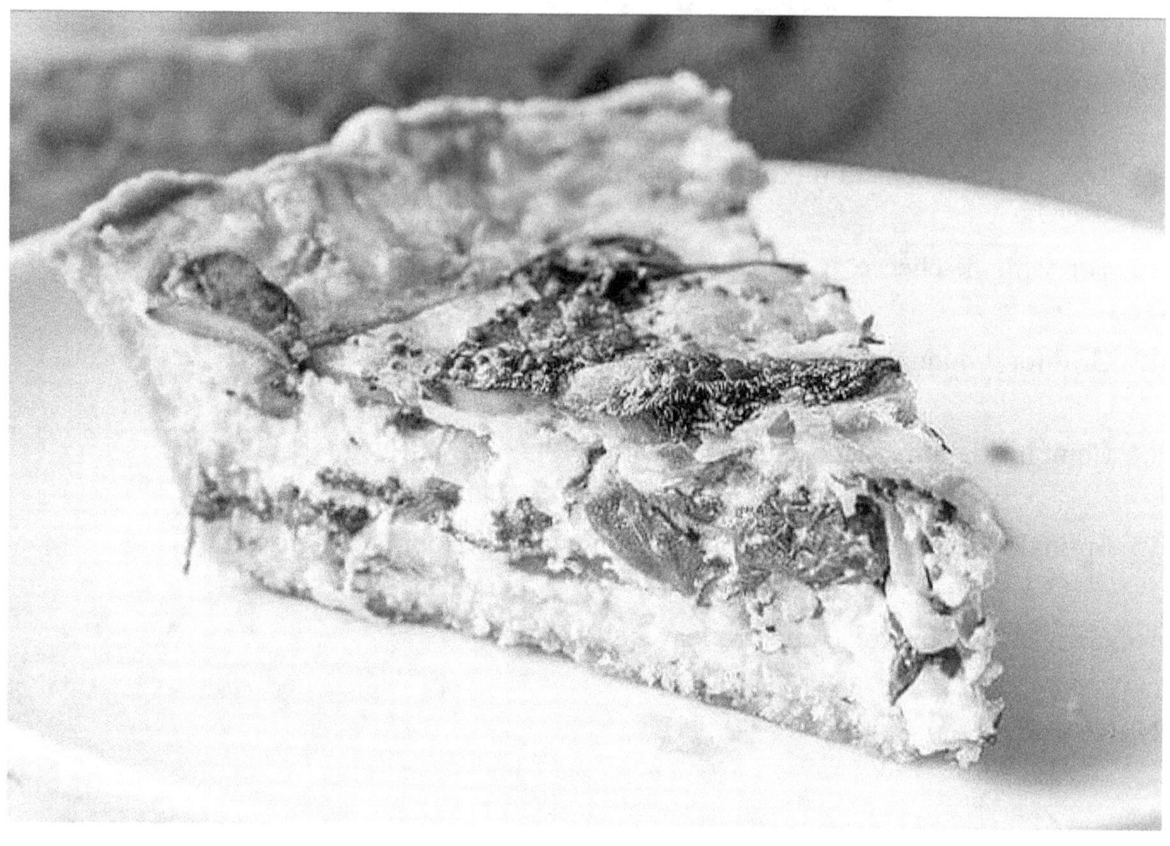

Healthy, delicious and best of all, fuss free! There's nothing more you can ask for from this incredible quiche loaded with fresh mushrooms, spinach and Gruyere cheese. Serve it with crusty bread or salad.

Serving Size: 6

Preparation Cooking Time: 1 hour and 5 minutes

Ingredients:

- 2 tablespoons olive oil
- 8 oz. mixed mushrooms
- 1 onion, chopped
- 1 tablespoon garlic, minced
- 8 cups spinach, chopped
- 6 eggs, beaten
- ¼ cup cream
- ¼ cup nonfat milk
- 1 tablespoon Dijon mustard
- Salt and pepper to taste
- 1 tablespoon thyme, chopped
- 1 cup Gruyere cheese, shredded

Instructions:

1. Preheat your oven to 375 degrees F.

2. Spray your pie pan with oil. Set aside.

3. Pour the oil into a pan over medium high heat.

4. Add the mushrooms and cook for 8 minutes.

5. Add the onion and garlic. Cook for 5 minutes.

6. Stir in the spinach, then cook for 2 minutes.

7. Remove from the stove.

8. In a bowl, mix the eggs, cream, milk, mustard, salt, pepper and thyme.

9. Stir in the mushroom and spinach mixture along with the cheese.

10. Spread the mixture to the baking pan.

11. Bake for 30 minutes.

12. Lastly, let sit for 10 minutes before slicing and serving.

Nutrients per Serving:

- *Calories 277*
- *Fat 20 g*
- *Saturated fat 8.2 g*
- *Carbohydrates 6.8 g*
- *Fiber 1.5 g*
- *Protein 17.1 g*
- *Cholesterol 220 mg*
- *Sugars 3 g*
- *Sodium 443 mg*
- *Potassium 289 mg*

Braised Brisket

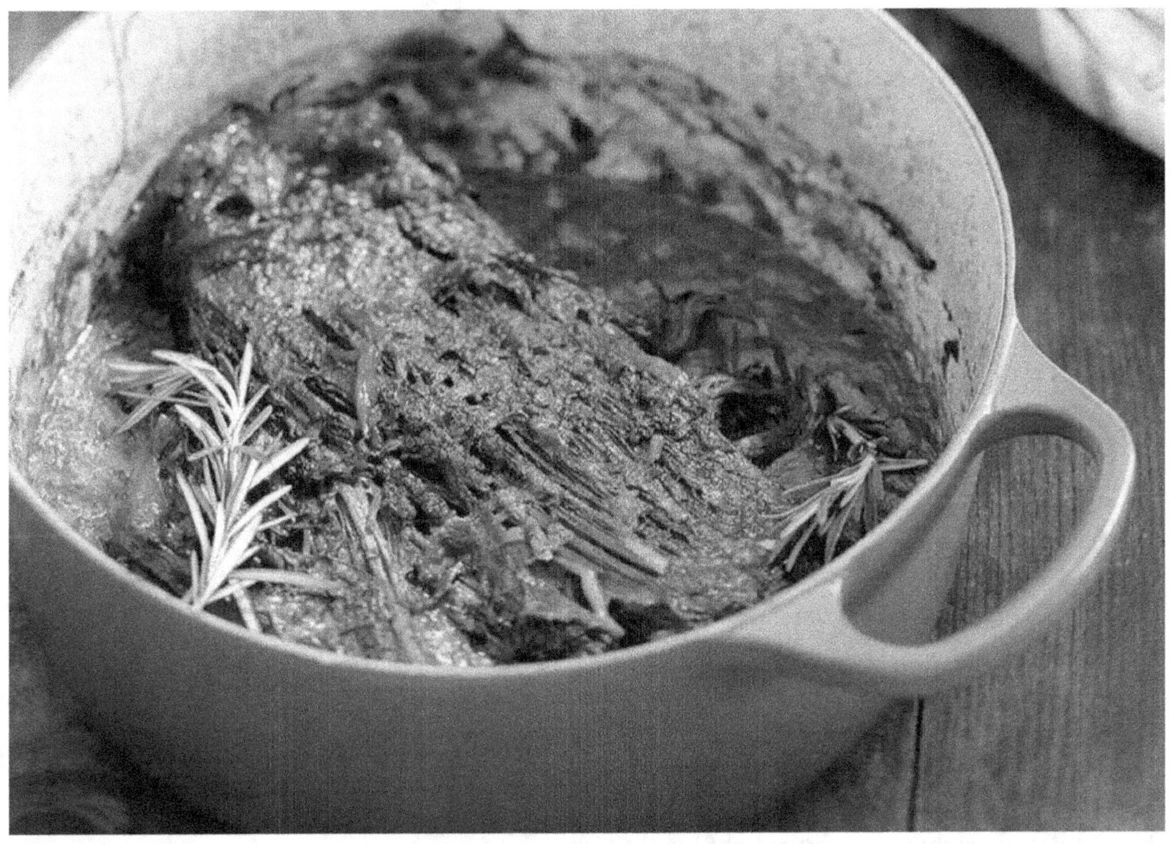

While this photo may not look as attractive or colorful as other dishes, don't make the mistake of thinking that it's nothing impressive. This braised brisket with dried fruits is packed with incredible flavors you can't believe.

Serving Size: 10

Preparation Cooking Time: 4 hours and 50 minutes

Ingredients:

- 3 star anise
- 1 teaspoon ground cinnamon
- 4 teaspoons ground sumac
- 4 teaspoons cocoa powder (unsweetened)
- 2 teaspoons red pepper flakes
- 4 lb. beef brisket, fat trimmed
- Salt to taste
- 2 tablespoons olive oil
- 4 white onions, sliced
- 8 cloves garlic, crushed and minced
- ¼ cup dried apricots
- ¼ cup dried cranberries
- ¼ cup prunes, pitted
- ¼ cup golden raisins
- 1 orange, sliced into wedges
- 4 cups reduced-sodium beef broth

Instructions:

1. Preheat your oven to 325 degrees F.

2. Grind the star anise using a grinder.

3. Transfer to a bowl. Mix with the cinnamon, sumac, cocoa powder and pepper.

4. Next, sprinkle both sides of the brisket with the salt and 2 tablespoons of the cinnamon mixture.

5. Pour the oil into a pot over high heat.

6. Cook the brisket for 4 minutes per side.

7. Transfer to a plate.

8. Reduce heat and add the onions.

9. Cook for 10 minutes, stirring often.

10. Add the remaining ingredients except the broth.

11. Stir in the remaining cinnamon mixture.

12. Cook for 3 minutes.

13. Pour in the broth and simmer.

14. Put the brisket back to the pot.

15. Cover and transfer to the oven.

16. Bake for 3 hours and 30 minutes.

17. Then, let the brisket rest for 10 minutes before slicing.

18. Lastly, serve with the sauce poured on top.

Nutrients per Serving:

- Calories 290
- *Fat 9.3 g*
- *Saturated fat 2.8 g*
- *Carbohydrates 15.7 g*
- *Fiber 2.2 g*
- *Protein 35.5 g*
- *Cholesterol 98 mg*
- *Sugars 10 g*
- *Sodium 320 mg*
- *Potassium 758 mg*

Baked Salmon with Radish Onions

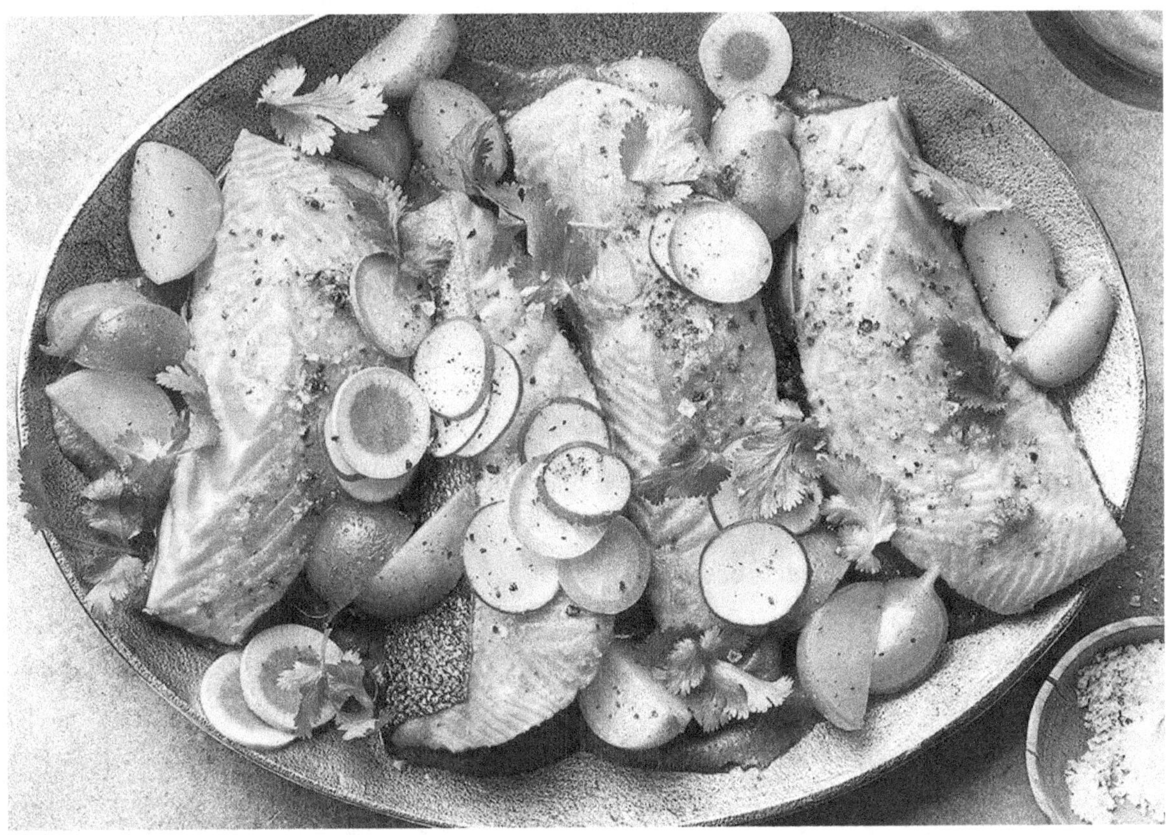

Pureed grilled onion creates amazing flavors for this baked salmon dish that's ready in less than an hour. Top with crunchy radish slices for best results.

Serving Size: 4

Preparation Cooking Time: 50 minutes

Ingredients:

- 2 onions, sliced
- 4 tablespoons olive oil, divided
- Salt and pepper to taste
- 1 teaspoon lemon zest
- 4 salmon fillets
- 6 radishes, sliced into rounds
- 1 teaspoon Old Bay seasoning
- ½ teaspoon sugar

Instructions:

1. Preheat your oven to 325 degrees F.

2. Put the pan over medium high heat.

3. Cook the onions for 15 minutes until a little charred.

4. Transfer to a bowl and cover.

5. In a bowl, combine half of the oil with the salt, pepper and lemon zest.

6. Pour 1 tablespoon oil into a pan.

7. Sprinkle the lemon zest mixture on both sides of the salmon.

8. Add the salmon to the pan.

9. Bake in the oven for 15 minutes.

10. Cook the radishes in the remaining oil in a pan over medium heat.

11. Set aside.

12. Add the charred onions, salt and sugar in a food processor.

13. Pulse until smooth.

14. Serve the salmon spread with the pureed onion and garnished with the radishes.

Nutrients per Serving:

- *Calories 324*
- *Fat 19.3 g*
- *Saturated fat 3.3 g*
- *Carbohydrates 7.4 g*
- *Fiber 1.8 g*
- *Protein 29.1 g*
- *Cholesterol 66 mg*
- *Sugars 3 g*
- *Sodium 718 mg*
- *Potassium 653 mg*

Chickpea Dumplings

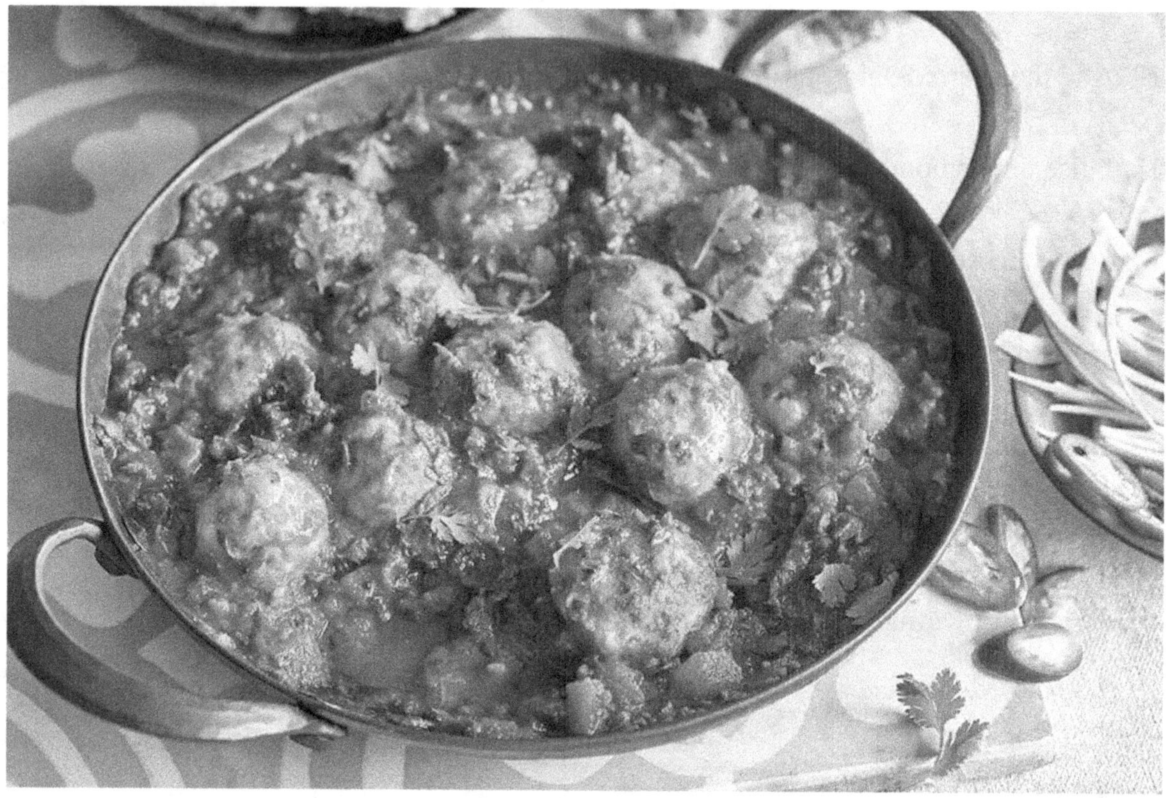

Do you love dumplings? Wait until you've tried this recipe that makes dumplings using chickpeas and soaking it in rich and creamy tomato sauce.

Serving Size: 4

Preparation Cooking Time: 45 minutes

Ingredients:

- 1 cup chickpea flour
- ¼ cup vegetable oil
- 1 onion, chopped
- ¼ cup low-fat plain yogurt
- ¼ cup jalapeño pepper, chopped
- 4 cups spinach, chopped and divided
- Salt to taste
- Cooking spray
- 1 teaspoon cumin seeds
- 2 teaspoons coriander seeds
- 1 teaspoon mustard seeds
- 1 tablespoon fresh ginger, minced
- 1 tablespoon curry powder
- 15 oz. canned tomato sauce
- 15 oz. canned diced tomatoes

Instructions:

1. First, in a large bowl, combine the chickpea flour, vegetable oil, onion, yogurt, jalapeño pepper, spinach and salt.

2. Form into dumplings.

3. Spray your skillet with oil.

4. Add the cumin, coriander and mustard seeds.

5. Cook for 30 seconds.

6. Stir in the rest of the ingredients.

7. Bring to a boil.

8. Add the dumplings to the sauce.

9. Lastly, cover and cook for 20 minutes or until tender.

Nutrients per Serving:

- *Calories 454*
- *Fat 29.2 g*
- *Saturated fat 2.3 g*
- *Carbohydrates 40.6 g*
- *Fiber 12.5 g*
- *Protein 12.3 g*
- *Cholesterol 2 mg*
- *Sugars 13 g*
- *Sodium 438 mg*
- *Potassium 805 mg*

Butternut Squash Soup

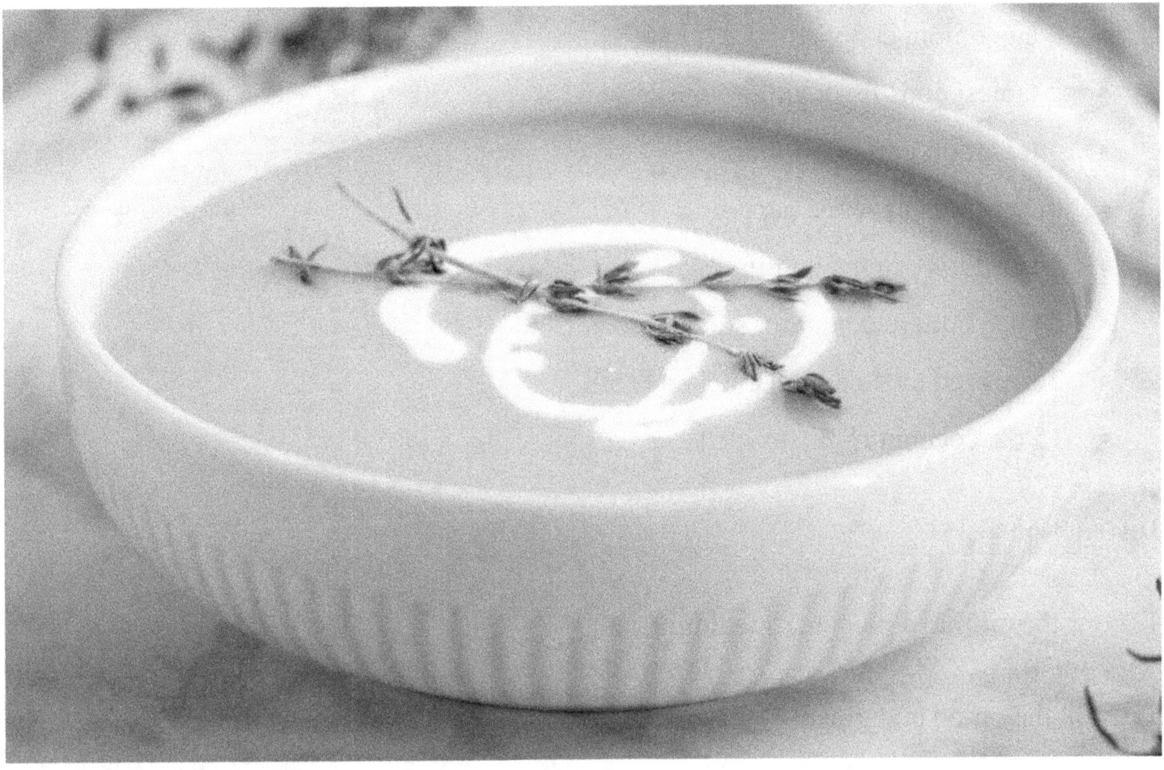

What makes this butternut squash soup more interesting is the addition of turmeric, cumin and ginger. The soup is best served with grilled cheese sandwich.

Serving Size: 4

Preparation Cooking Time: 45 minutes

Ingredients:

- 1 tablespoon coconut oil
- 1 cup onion, chopped
- 2 tablespoons fresh ginger, minced
- 1 teaspoon ground turmeric
- ¼ teaspoon cayenne pepper
- 1 teaspoon ground cumin
- 5 cups butternut squash, sliced into cubes
- 2 cups reduced-sodium chicken broth
- 15 oz. coconut milk, divided

Instructions:

1. Pour the oil into a pan over medium heat.

2. Cook the onion and ginger for 3 minutes.

3. Stir in the turmeric, cayenne pepper and cumin.

4. Cook while stirring for 30 seconds.

5. Add the squash, broth and coconut milk.

6. Cook for 20 minutes.

7. Transfer the soup to a blender.

8. Pulse until smooth.

9. Reheat before serving.

Nutrients per Serving:

- *Calories 419*
- *Fat 23.1 g*
- *Saturated fat 10.6 g*
- *Carbohydrates 43.3 g*
- *Fiber 8.4 g*
- *Protein 13.5 g*
- *Cholesterol 26 mg*
- *Sugars 10 g*
- *Sodium 827 mg*
- *Potassium 623 mg*

Pesto Chicken Pizza with Cauliflower Salad

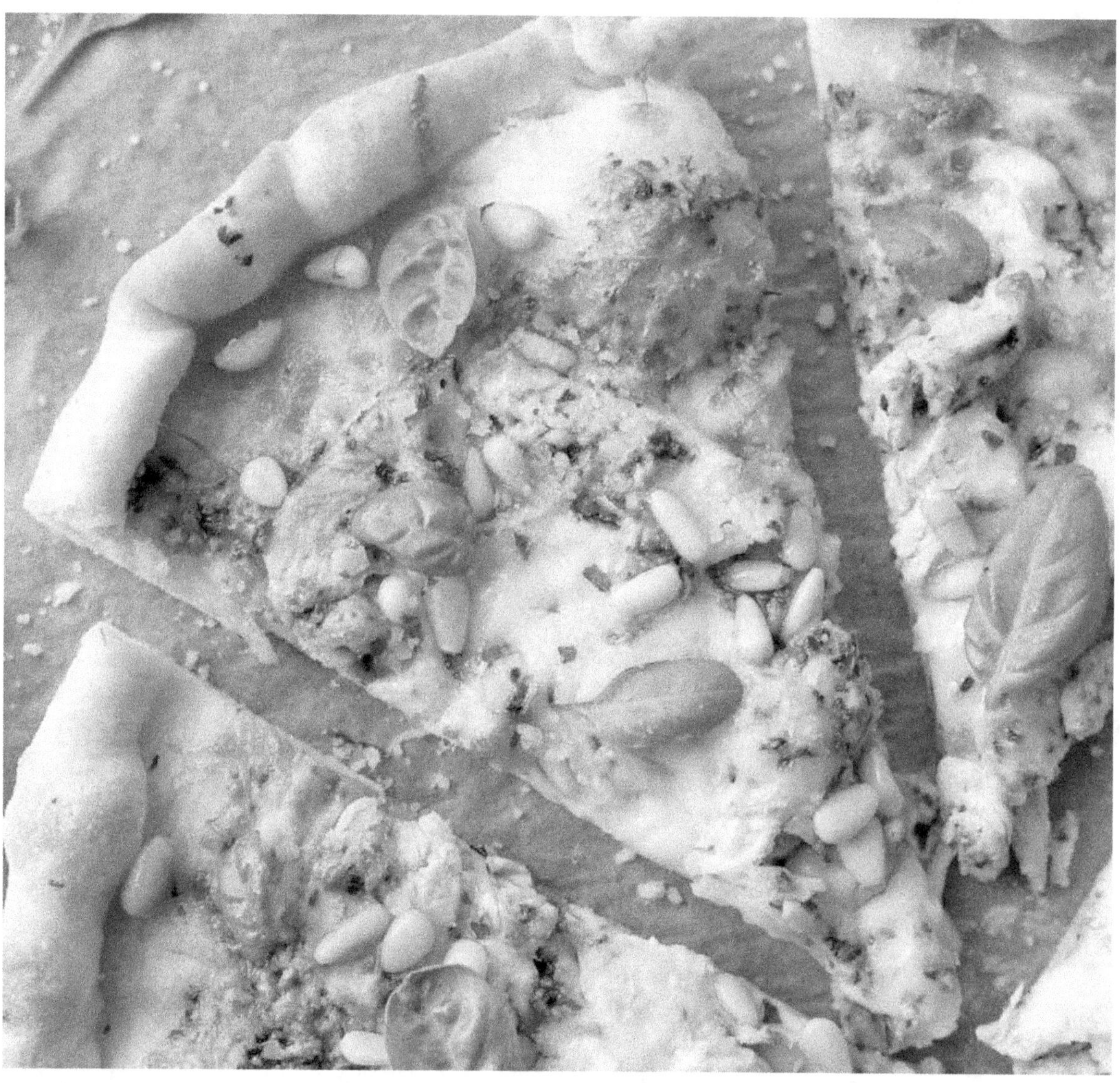

This is nothing like the other pizzas you've tried before. What makes this one different is that the crust is made using cauliflower. You're in for a sweet surprise.

Serving Size: 4

Preparation Cooking Time: 30 minutes

Ingredients:

- 2 chicken thigh fillets
- Salt and pepper to taste
- 12 oz. cauliflower pizza crust
- ¼ cup pesto
- 1 cup mozzarella cheese
- 1 head iceberg lettuce, chopped
- 1 cup cherry tomatoes, sliced in half
- 1 cup cauliflower, chopped
- 1 oz. pepperoni, chopped

Dressing

- ¾ cup red-wine vinegar
- 5 tablespoons water
- 1 ½ tablespoons sugar
- 1 tablespoon Dijon mustard
- 1 clove garlic
- 2 teaspoons dried basil
- 2 teaspoons dried oregano
- Salt and pepper to taste
- 1 ¾ cups olive oil

Instructions:

1. Preheat your oven to 425 degrees F.

2. Add the chicken to a baking pan.

3. Next, sprinkle both sides with the salt and pepper.

4. Bake in the oven for 15 minutes.

5. Shred the chicken.

6. Prepare the crust according to the directions in the package.

7. Spread the pesto on top of the crust.

8. Top with the mozzarella and shredded chicken.

9. Bake until the cheese has melted.

10. In a bowl, mix the lettuce, tomatoes, cauliflower and pepperoni.

11. Then, add all the dressing ingredients to a food processor.

12. Pulse until smooth.

13. Toss the salad in the dressing.

14. Serve the pizza with the salad.

Nutrients per Serving:

- *Calories 514*
- *Fat 38.4 g*
- *Saturated fat 8.9 g*
- *Carbohydrates 25.1 g*
- *Fiber 4.3 g*
- *Protein 18 g*
- *Cholesterol 46 mg*
- *Sugars 8 g*
- *Sodium 731 mg*
- *Potassium 551 mg*

Chicken Steak with Gravy

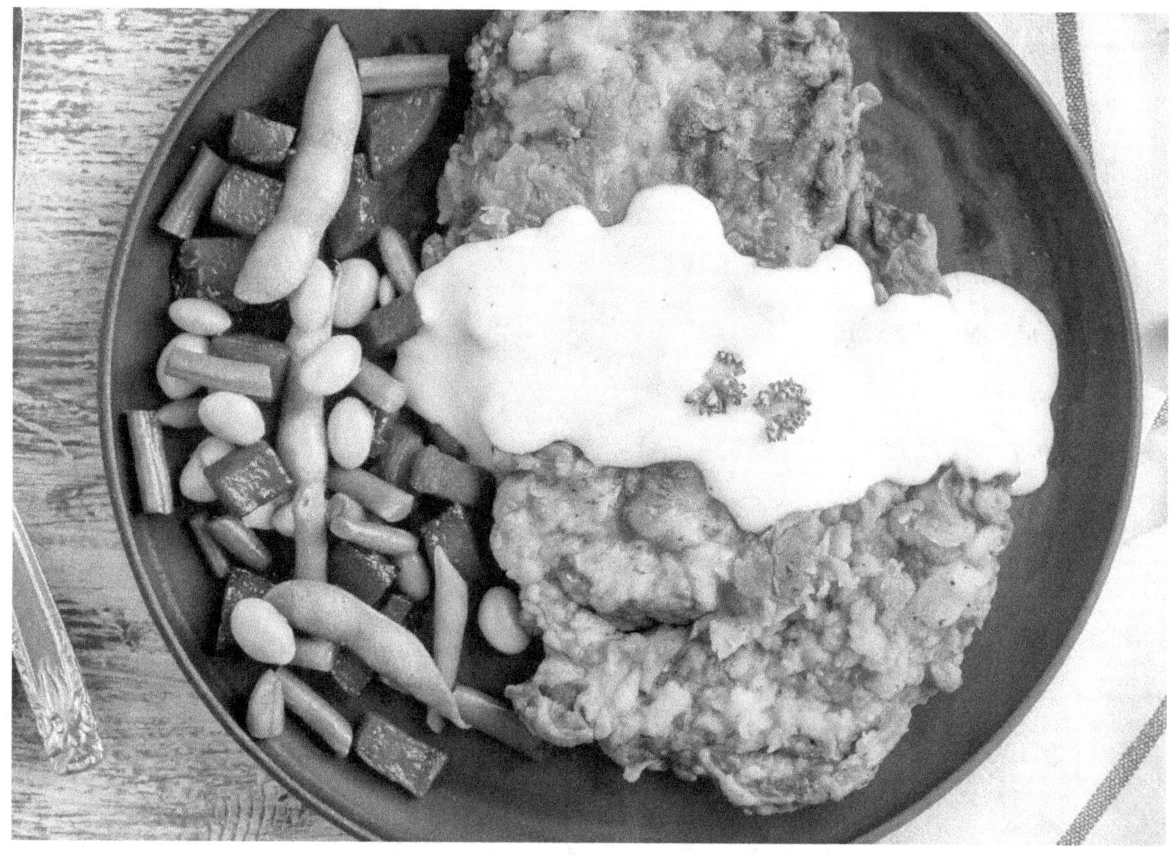

This baked version of crunchy chicken steak lets you enjoy your favorite dish without having to worry too much about grease and fat. Pour gravy on top and serve with steamed green beans.

Serving Size: 4

Preparation Cooking Time: 30 minutes

Ingredients:

- 1 lb. chicken thigh fillet, sliced into strips
- ¼ cup all-purpose flour
- ½ teaspoon garlic powder
- 1 tablespoon Parmesan cheese, grated
- ⅛ teaspoon cayenne pepper
- ¼ teaspoon ground coriander
- ¼ teaspoon ground cumin
- Salt to taste
- ¼ cup low-fat buttermilk
- 1 egg white, beaten
- 1 cup cornflakes, crushed
- 1 tablespoon butter
- ¾ cup nonfat milk
- Pinch ground nutmeg
- Steamed green beans

Instructions:

1. Preheat your oven to 425 degrees F.

2. Spray your baking pan with oil.

3. In a bowl, mix the flour, garlic powder, Parmesan cheese, cayenne pepper, ground coriander, ground cumin and salt.

4. In another bowl, combine the low-fat buttermilk and egg white.

5. Add the crushed cornflakes to the third bowl.

6. Dip the chicken strips in the first, second and third bowls.

7. Arrange in a baking pan.

8. Next, bake for 20 minutes or until golden and crispy.

9. In a pan, simmer butter milk and nutmeg.

10. Then, pour the gravy on top of the chicken.

11. Serve with the steamed green beans.

Nutrients per Serving:

- *Calories 279*
- *Fat 6.5 g*
- *Saturated fat 3.2 g*
- *Carbohydrates 22.8 g*
- *Fiber 0.9 g*
- *Protein 31.5 g*
- *Cholesterol 75 mg*
- *Sugars 4 g*
- *Sodium 627 mg*
- *Potassium 518 mg*

Open-Faced Eggplant Sandwich

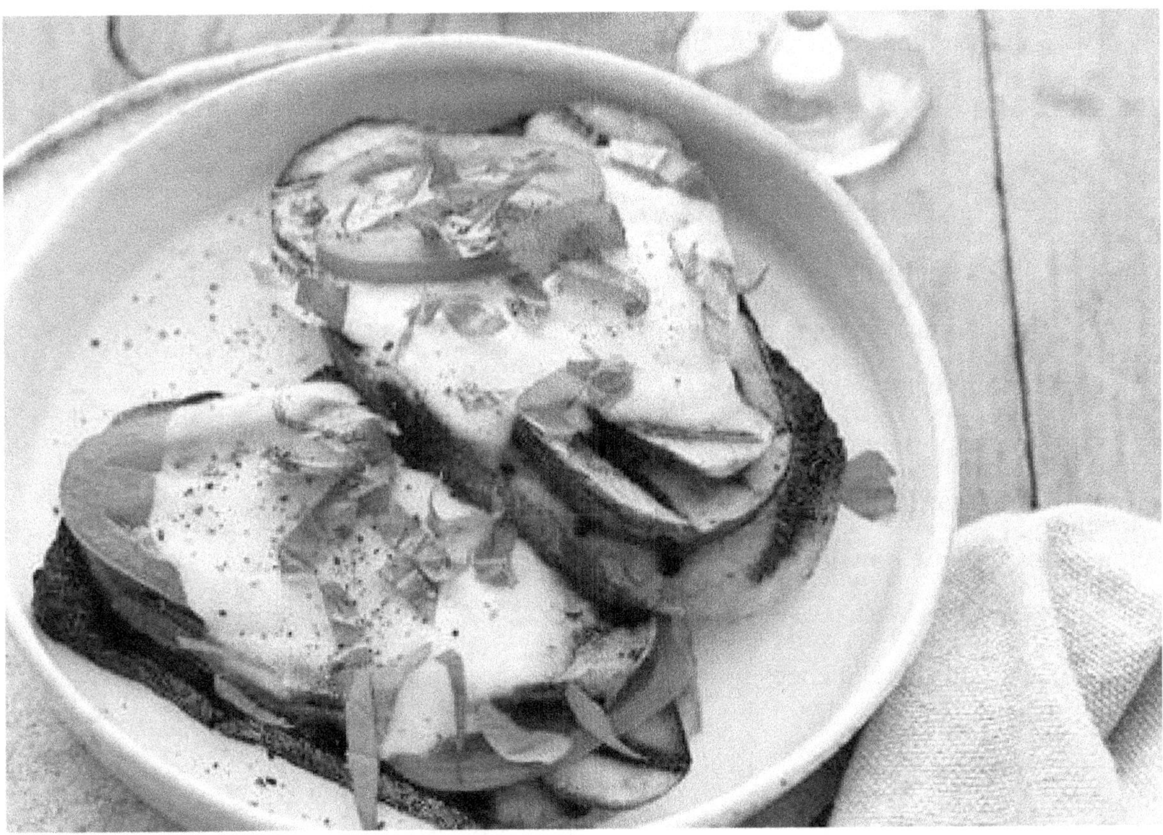

This is a combination of your two favorites: eggplant Parmesan and sandwich. Here's how to create this beautiful and delicious snack without the fuss.

Serving Size: 2

Preparation Cooking Time: 1 hour

Ingredients:

- ½ teaspoon olive oil
- ½ cup panko breadcrumbs, divided
- 2 egg whites, beaten and divided
- 2 tablespoons Parmesan cheese, grated and divided
- Pepper to taste
- 4 slices eggplant
- ¼ teaspoon dried parsley flakes
- Cooking spray
- 8 oz. lean ground beef
- ½ cup marinara sauce
- Pinch garlic powder
- 1 cup arugula
- ¼ cup mozzarella cheese

Instructions:

1. Preheat your oven to 375 degrees F.

2. Coat your baking pan with olive oil.

3. Add 1 egg white to a dish.

4. Stir in 5 tablespoons breadcrumbs and half of the Parmesan cheese.

5. Add the pepper and parsley flakes. Mix well.

6. Next, dip the eggplant slices in the egg whites and coat with the breadcrumbs.

7. Place on a baking sheet.

8. Spray with oil.

9. Next, bake for 30 minutes or until golden and crispy.

10. In a bowl, combine the ground beef with the remaining breadcrumbs, remaining Parmesan cheese, pepper, garlic powder and remaining egg white.

11. Mix and form patties from this mixture.

12. Then, grill the patties for 5 minutes per side.

13. Top each of the eggplant with the patty and pour with the marinara sauce.

14. Sprinkle with the arugula and cheese.

15. Bake until the cheese has melted.

Nutrients per Serving:

- *Calories 344*
- *Fat 12.1 g*
- *Saturated fat 5.1 g*
- *Carbohydrates 19.9 g*
- *Fiber 2.8 g*
- *Protein 36.4 g*
- *Cholesterol 82 mg*
- *Sugars 6 g*
- *Sodium 580 mg*
- *Potassium 613 mg*

Cauliflower Grilled Cheese Sandwich Tower

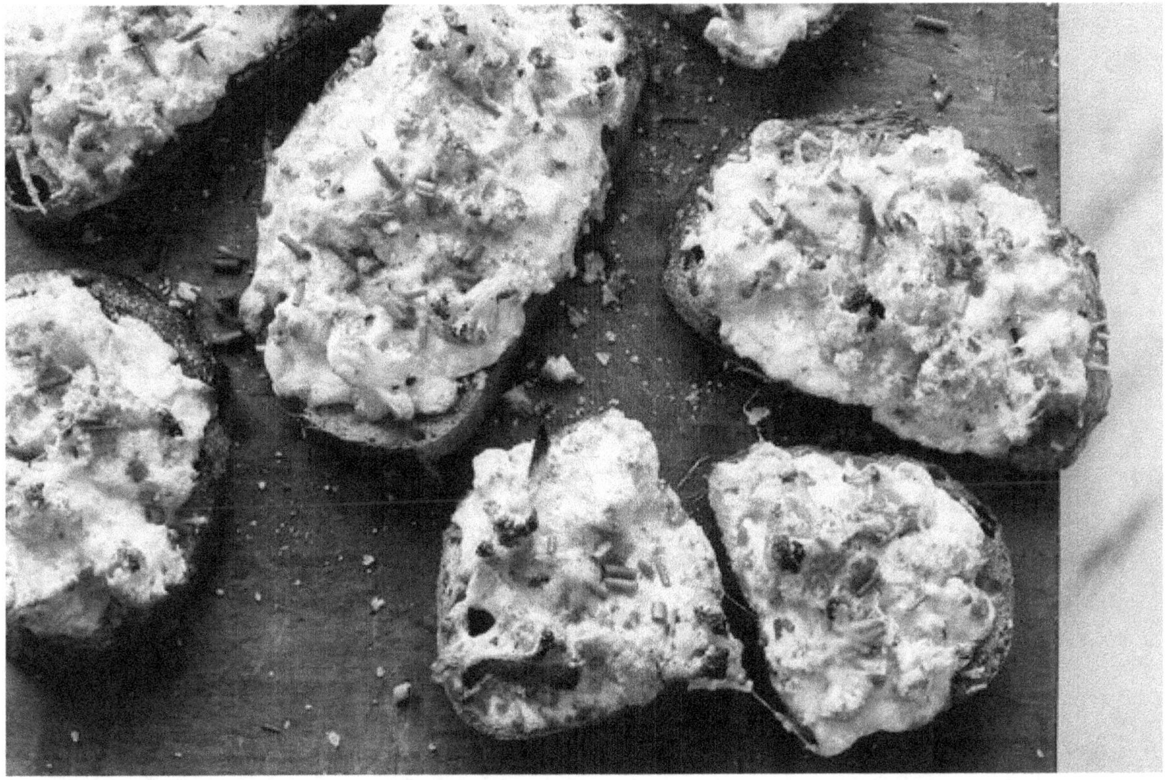

If you're looking for something heavy to fill you up, here's one that won't wreak havoc with your healthy diet. This is a sandwich tower loaded with cheese and cauliflower.

Serving Size: 4

Preparation Cooking Time: 50 minutes

Ingredients:

- 6 cups cauliflower florets
- 2 tablespoons oil
- Salt and pepper to taste
- 1 teaspoon dried oregano
- 1 ¼ cups cheddar cheese, shredded
- 2 tablespoons butter, softened
- 8 slices whole-wheat sourdough bread
- 8 teaspoons sun-dried tomatoes, chopped

Instructions:

1. Preheat your oven to 425 degrees F.

2. Spray your baking pan with oil.

3. Toss the cauliflower in oil and season with the salt and pepper.

4. Transfer to the baking pan and roast for 15 minutes.

5. In a bowl, mix the oregano and cheddar.

6. Spread the butter on one side of the sourdough bread.

7. Top with the cheese mixture, tomatoes and cauliflower.

8. Repeat the layers until you've used up all the bread slices and ingredients.

9. Bake in the oven for 3 minutes.

Nutrients per Serving:

- *Calories 488*
- *Fat 27.6 g*
- *Saturated fat 11.5 g*
- *Carbohydrates 40.4 g*
- *Fiber 7.6 g*
- *Protein 17.5 g*
- *Cholesterol 50 mg*
- *Sugars 7 g*
- *Sodium 832 mg*
- *Potassium 583 mg*

Spicy Salmon with Apricots

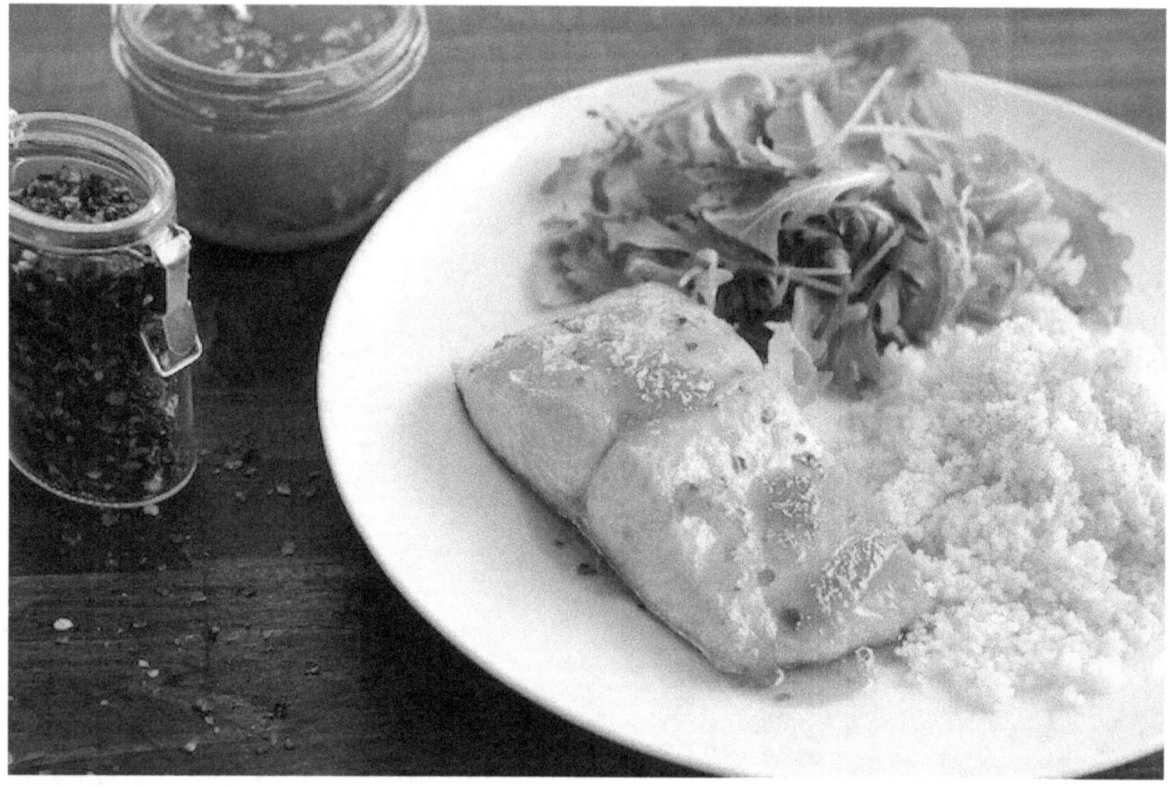

A 30-minute salmon dish that won't disappoint your taste buds—this is a definite must-try.

Serving Size: 4

Preparation Cooking Time: 30 minutes

Ingredients:

- ¼ cup apricot preserves
- ½ cup apricot nectar
- 3 tablespoons scallions, chopped
- Salt and pepper to taste
- ½ teaspoon dried oregano
- 8 dried apricots, sliced in half and soaked in hot water for 1 hour
- 2 teaspoons hot pepper sauce
- 4 salmon fillets
- 1 tablespoon olive oil

Instructions:

1. Add the apricot preserves and nectar in a pan over medium heat.

2. Stir in the scallions, salt, pepper and oregano.

3. Simmer for 8 minutes or until thickened.

4. Reserve ¼ cup of the sauce.

5. Next, add the dried apricots and pepper sauce to the remaining mixture in the pan.

6. Remove from heat.

7. Then, season the fish with the salt and pepper.

8. Grill for 3 to 4 minutes per side, brushing with the reserved sauce.

9. Pour the sauce from the pan on top of the fish and serve.

Nutrients per Serving:

- *Calories 304*
- *Fat 8.4 g*
- *Saturated fat 1.3 g*
- *Carbohydrates 27.1 g*
- *Fiber 1.6 g*
- *Protein 29.1 g*
- *Cholesterol 73 mg*
- *Sugars 16 g*
- *Sodium 260 mg*
- *Potassium 637 mg*

Veggie Lasagna

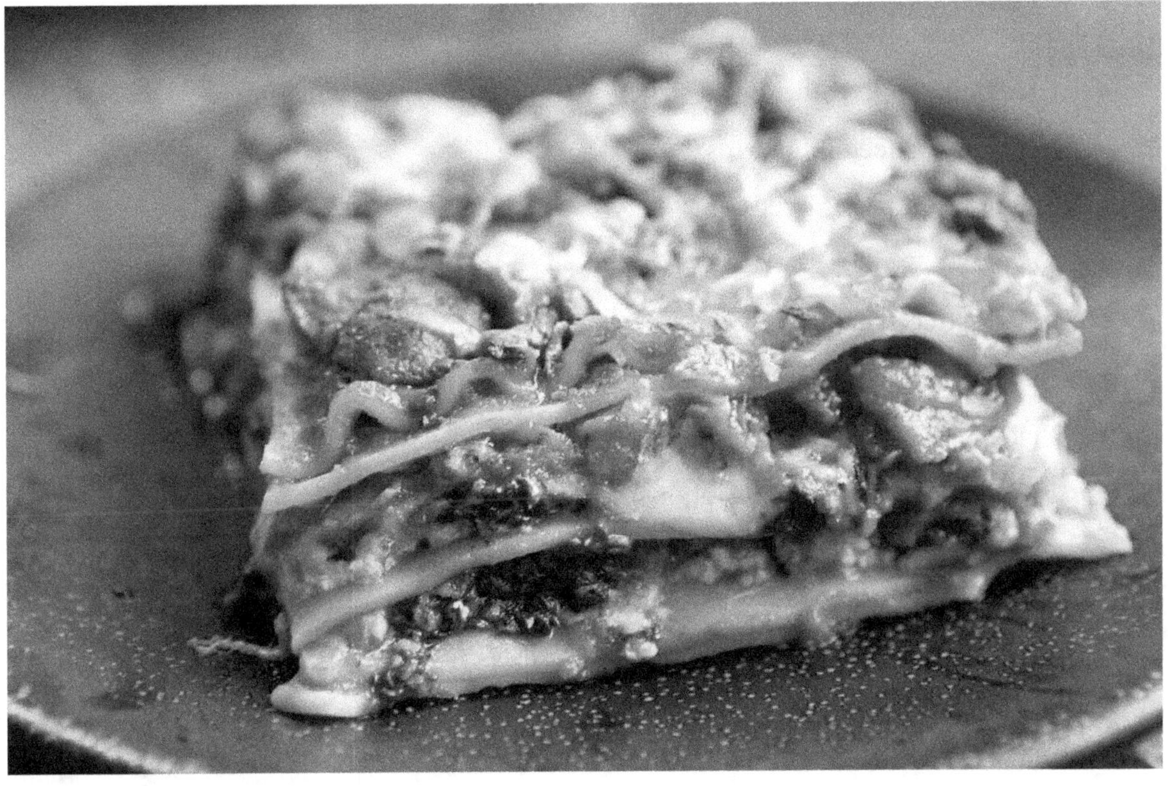

This lasagna recipe is as delicious as it is colorful. You won't only have fun preparing it, you'll also enjoy the fact that it's tasty and healthy.

Serving Size: 8

Preparation Cooking Time: 6 hours

Ingredients:

- 9 cooked lasagna noodles
- 6 cups broccoli florets
- 1 red bell pepper, sliced into strips
- 1 zucchini, sliced into strips
- 1 summer squash, sliced
- 2 eggs
- 15 oz. reduced-fat ricotta cheese
- 16 oz. reduced-fat cottage cheese
- 3 cloves garlic, crushed and minced
- 2 tablespoons fresh thyme, chopped
- ½ cup fresh basil leaves, chopped
- Salt and pepper to taste
- 2 cups mozzarella cheese, shredded and divided

Instructions:

1. Spray your baking pan with oil. Set aside

2. Pour 2 cups water into a pot.

3. Add a steamer basket inside.

4. Steam the vegetables for 7 minutes or until tender but still crispy.

5. Remove from the stove.

6. Next, in a bowl, beat the eggs and stir in the rest of the ingredients except the mozzarella.

7. Arrange the lasagna noodles in a single layer.

8. Top with the cheese mixture and then with the veggies.

9. Repeat the layers.

10. Top with the mozzarella cheese.

11. Lastly, bake in the oven at 375 degrees for 50 minutes.

Nutrients per Serving:

- *Calories 296*
- *Fat 7.4 g*
- *Saturated fat 3.9 g*
- *Carbohydrates 31.7 g*
- *Fiber 3.7 g*
- *Protein 26.6 g*
- *Cholesterol 86 mg*
- *Sugars 8 g*
- *Sodium 723 mg*
- *Potassium 557 mg*

Salmon Loaf

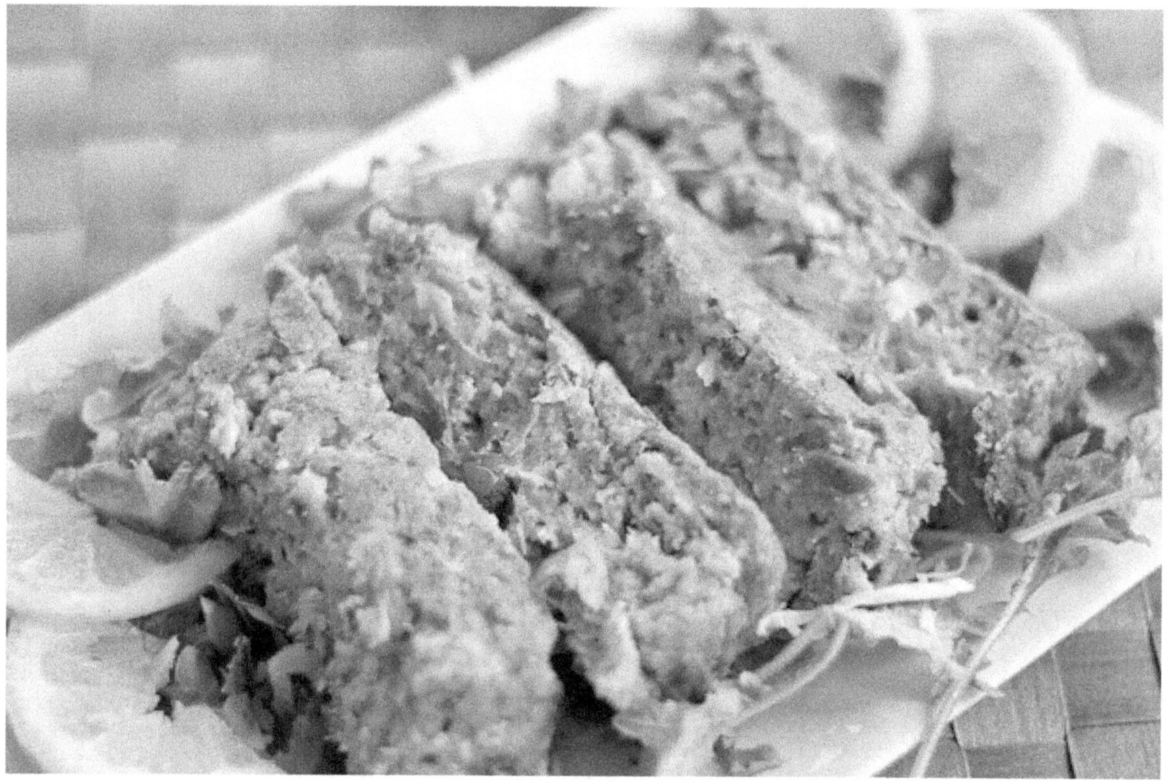

This salmon loaf is very easy to make but so impressive that friends are going to think you spent a lot of effort preparing this.

Serving Size: 6

Preparation Cooking Time: 1 hour and 30 minutes

Ingredients:

- 15 oz. canned salmon flakes
- 1 onion, chopped
- 1 stalk celery, chopped
- 2 tablespoons parsley, chopped
- 1 tablespoon fresh dill, chopped
- ¼ cup breadcrumbs
- 1 cup cooked barley
- Pepper to taste
- 2 tablespoons freshly squeezed lemon juice
- 2 eggs, beaten
- Cooking spray
- ½ cup peas, cooked
- 2 ½ teaspoons cornstarch
- 1 cup nonfat milk
- Lemon zest
- Salt to taste

Instructions:

1. Preheat your oven to 350 degrees F.

2. Combine the salmon flakes, onion, celery, parsley, dill, breadcrumbs, barley and pepper in a bowl.

3. Stir in the eggs.

4. Mix well.

5. Cover your loaf pan with foil and spray with oil.

6. Press the mixture into the loaf pan.

7. Bake for 1 hour.

8. Let stand for 10 minutes before slicing.

9. In a pan, combine the remaining ingredients.

10. Cook for 2 minutes.

11. Serve the salmon slices with the creamy peas.

Nutrients per Serving:

- *Calories 275*
- *Fat 6.9 g*
- *Saturated fat 1.3 g*
- *Carbohydrates 17 g*
- *Fiber 2 g*
- *Protein 36.4 g*
- *Cholesterol 109 mg*
- *Sugars 4 g*
- *Sodium 747 mg*
- *Potassium 608 mg*

Steak Burgers

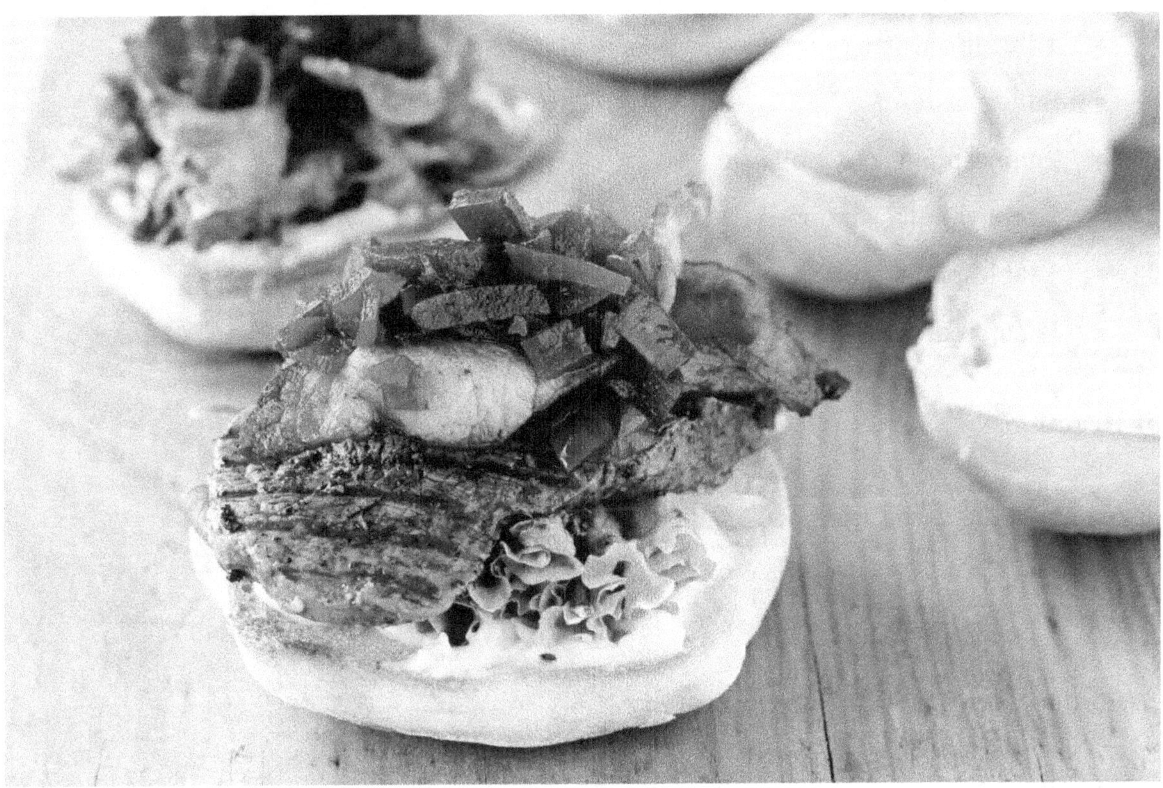

What makes this burger different from the others you've tried is that this one is not made with ground beef but with chopped sirloin steak. Taste the difference yourself.

Serving Size: 4

Preparation Cooking Time: 40 minutes

Ingredients:

- 1 clove garlic, grated
- 1 lb. sirloin steak, chopped
- Salt to taste
- 2 tablespoons olive oil
- 2 fennel bulbs, chopped
- 1 tablespoon fresh sage, chopped
- ¼ cup red-wine vinegar

Instructions:

1. Combine the garlic, chopped steak and salt in a bowl.

2. Mix well.

3. Form 4 patties from the mixture.

4. Pour the oil into a pan over medium heat.

5. Cook the burgers for 4 minutes per side.

6. Transfer the burgers to a plate.

7. Add the fennel to the pan and cook for 3 minutes.

8. Stir in the remaining ingredients.

9. Season with the salt.

10. Cook for 3 minutes.

11. Serve the burgers with the fennel.

Nutrients per Serving:

- *Calories 321*
- *Fat 18.8 g*
- *Saturated fat 5.7 g*
- *Carbohydrates 9.7 g*
- *Fiber 4 g*
- *Protein 27.6 g*
- *Cholesterol 81 mg*
- *Sugars 5 g*
- *Sodium 560 mg*
- *Potassium 879 mg*

Chicken Avocado Sandwich

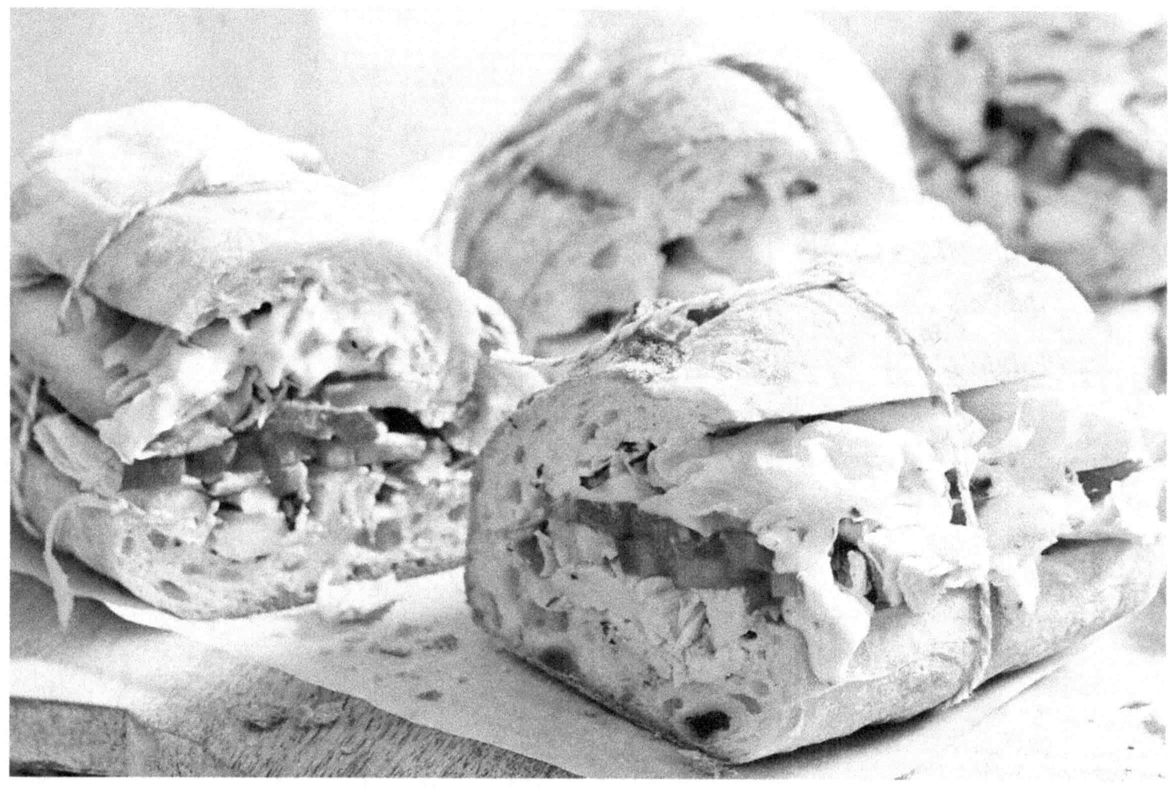

This recipe is inspired from the Venezuelan sandwich recipe, in which corn rolls are stuffed with filling and fried crispy. In this recipe, the sandwich is loaded with delicious chicken and avocado salad.

Serving Size: 4

Preparation Cooking Time: 50 minutes

Ingredients:

- 12 oz. chicken breast fillet
- 1 ¼ cups all-purpose flour
- Salt to taste
- 1 ½ cups water
- 1 tablespoon oil
- 1 cup ripe avocado, cubed
- 2 tablespoons lime juice
- ¼ cup fat-free plain yogurt
- 2 scallions, chopped
- Pepper to taste

Instructions:

1. Preheat your oven to 350 degrees F.

2. Add the chicken to a saucepan.

3. Cover the chicken with cold water.

4. Put the pan over medium high heat.

5. Bring to a boil.

6. Reduce heat and simmer for 15 minutes.

7. Transfer the chicken to a plate.

8. Combine the flour and salt.

9. Gradually add the water.

10. Mix until you form smooth dough.

11. Knead the dough for 1 minute.

12. Shape into a ball.

13. Cover the dough with towel and let sit for 5 minutes.

14. Divide it into 4 pieces.

15. Form a disk shape from each piece.

16. Pour the oil into a pan over medium heat.

17. Cook the dough for 3 minutes per side.

18. Add the pan to the oven.

19. Bake for 15 minutes.

20. Shred the cooked chicken and add to a bowl.

21. Add the avocado and mash.

22. Stir in the remaining ingredients. Mix well.

23. Slice each of the bread to form a pocket.

24. Stuff each one with the chicken and avocado salad.

Nutrients per Serving:

- *Calories 426*
- *Fat 13.2 g*
- *Saturated fat 1.8 g*
- *Carbohydrates 50 g*
- *Fiber 3.6 g*
- *Protein 25.8 g*
- *Cholesterol 63 mg*
- *Sugars 1 g*
- *Sodium 344 mg*
- *Potassium 580 mg*

Chickpea Quinoa Salad

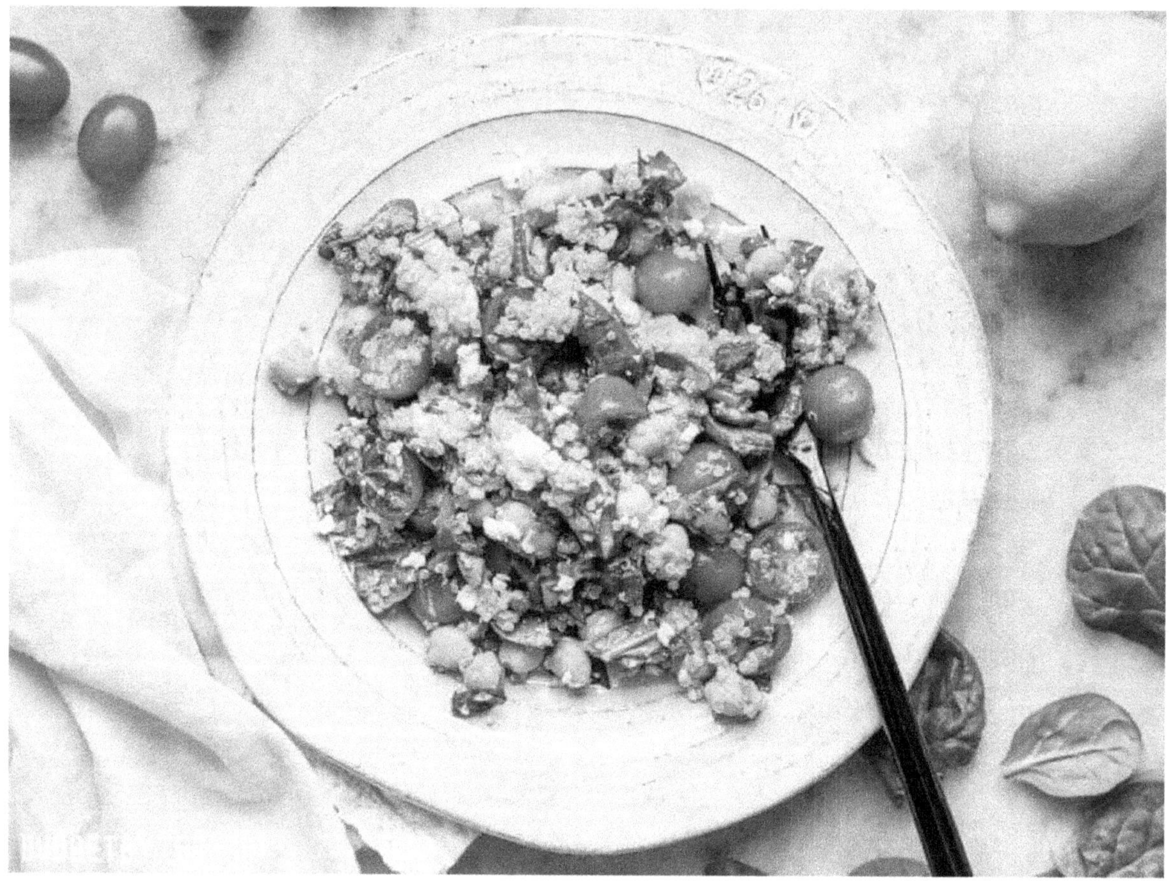

When you're feeling low, this is one dish that can boost your mood and pump your energy—protein packed salad loaded with tasty quinoa, avocado and vegetables.

Serving Size: 2

Preparation Cooking Time: 30 minutes

Ingredients:

- ⅔ cup water
- ⅓ cup quinoa
- Salt to taste
- 1 clove garlic, crushed
- 3 tablespoons olive oil
- 3 tablespoons freshly squeezed lemon juice
- 2 teaspoons freshly grated lemon zest
- Pepper to taste
- ½ avocado, sliced into cubes
- 1 carrot, shredded
- 1 cup chickpeas, rinsed and drained
- 4 cups baby kale
- 4 cup baby spinach

Instructions:

1. Add the water to a pan over medium heat.

2. Bring to a boil.

3. Add the quinoa.

4. Reduce heat and simmer for 15 minutes.

5. Fluff the quinoa with a fork.

6. Let cool and set aside.

7. Add the salt to the garlic.

8. Mash to form a paste.

9. Next, transfer to a bowl and stir in the olive oil, lemon juice, lemon zest and pepper.

10. Take 3 tablespoons of this mixture and reserve for later use.

11. Then, add the avocado, carrots and chickpeas to the remaining dressing.

12. Toss to combine.

13. Let sit for 5 minutes.

14. Stir in the quinoa.

15. Toss gently.

16. Add the leafy greens in a serving bowl.

17. Drizzle with the reserved dressing.

18. Spread the quinoa mixture on top.

Nutrients per Serving:

- *Calories 501*
- *Fat 31.5 g*
- *Saturated fat 4.3 g*
- *Carbohydrates 47.3 g*
- *Fiber 12.9 g*
- *Protein 12 g*
- *Cholesterol 30 mg*
- *Sugars 7 g*
- *Sodium 349 mg*
- *Potassium 844 mg*

Meatloaf

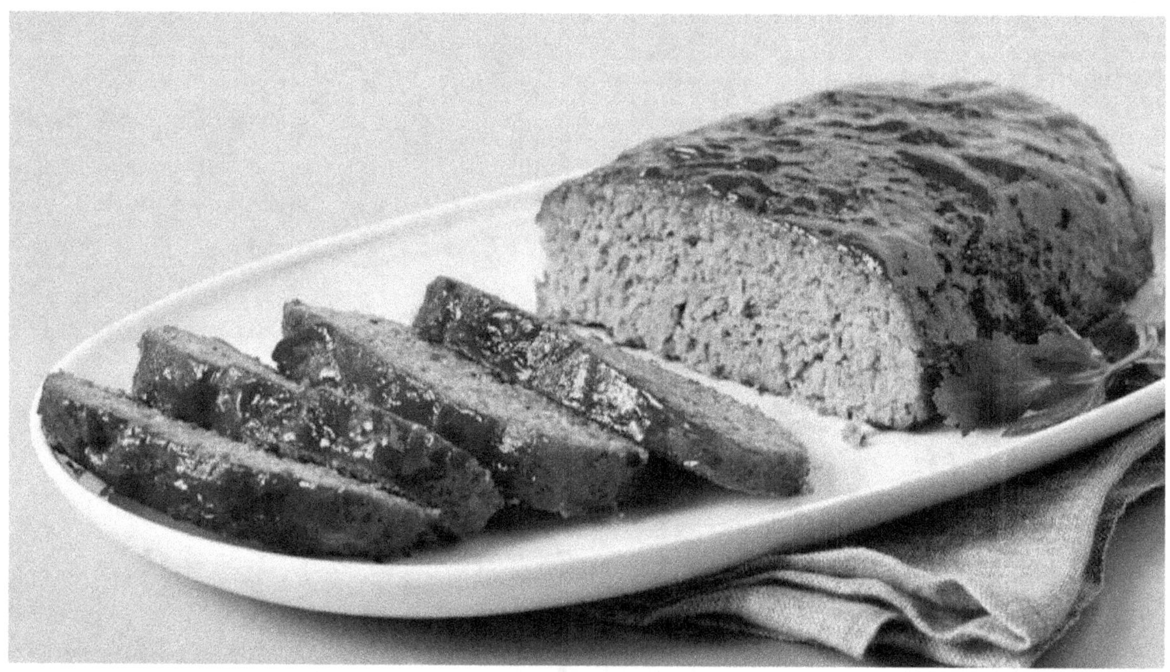

Oats, garlic and mushrooms pack in more nutrients and of course, enticing flavors to your regular meatloaf. Serve this with rice, bread or salad.

Serving Size: 6

Preparation Cooking Time: 1 hour and 40 minutes

Ingredients:

- ½ cup quick-cooking oats
- 1 ½ cups cremini mushrooms
- 1 tablespoon olive oil
- ½ cup onion, chopped
- 6 cloves garlic, crushed and minced
- 1 ½ lb. lean ground beef
- ½ cup green bell pepper, chopped
- 2 tablespoons cider vinegar
- 1 egg, beaten
- 1 tablespoon Dijon mustard
- Salt and pepper to taste
- 1 tablespoon Worcestershire sauce
- ¼ cup ketchup
- Cooking spray

Instructions:

1. Preheat your oven to 350 degrees F.

2. Add the oats to a food processor.

3. Pulse until fully ground.

4. Transfer the oats to a bowl and set aside.

5. Add the mushrooms to the food processor and pulse 10 times.

6. Pour the oil into a pan over medium heat.

7. Cook the onion, garlic and bell pepper for 3 minutes.

8. Stir in the mushrooms and cook for 4 minutes.

9. Pour in the vinegar and cook for 2 minutes.

10. Next, remove from heat and let cool for 10 minutes.

11. Add the mushrooms to the oats.

12. Stir in the remaining ingredients except the ketchup.

13. Mix gently.

14. Spray your loaf pan with oil.

15. Press the mixture into the loaf pan.

16. Brush the ketchup on top.

17. Bake in the oven for 1 hour.

18. Let cool before slicing and serving.

Nutrients per Serving:

- *Calories 255*
- *Fat 10.1 g*
- *Saturated fat 3.3 g*
- *Carbohydrates 12.3 g*
- *Fiber 1.5 g*
- *Protein 27.6 g*
- *Cholesterol 101 mg*
- *Sugars 4 g*
- *Sodium 349 mg*
- *Potassium 600 mg*

Salmon with Sorrel

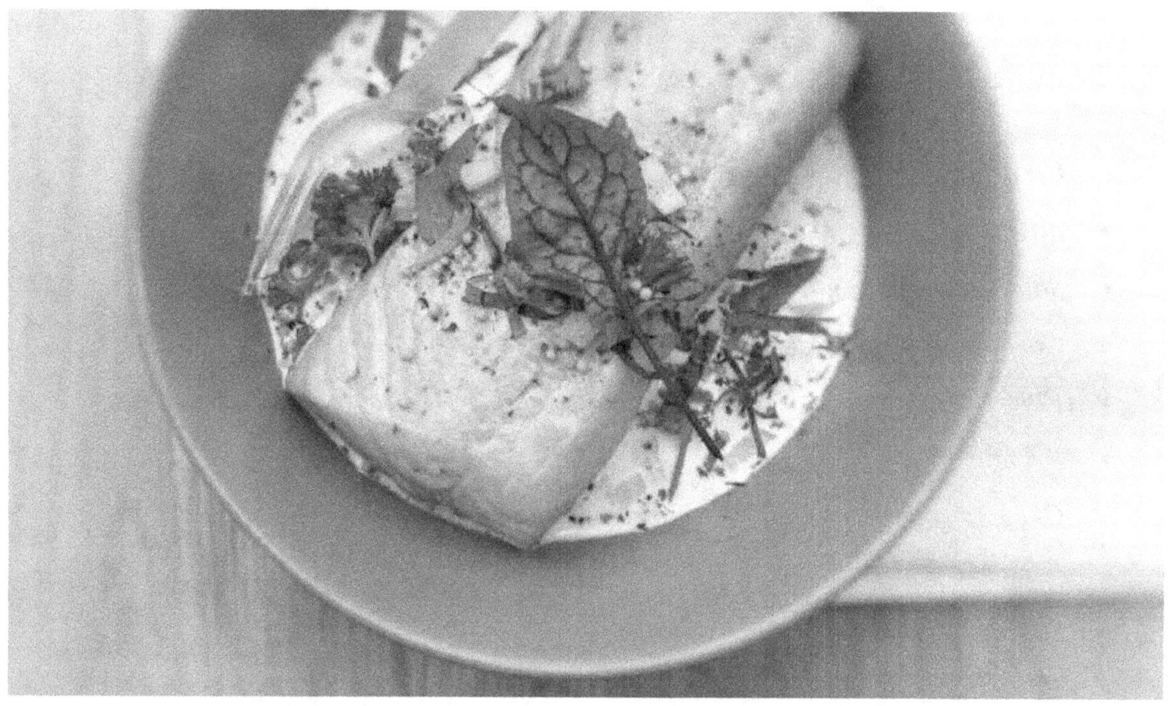

Sorrel, which is known for its lemon flavor, can up the ante of your regular salmon dish. This can be a marvelous addition to your weekly menu.

Serving Size: 4

Preparation Cooking Time: 45 minutes

Ingredients:

- ½ cup cold water
- 4 cups sorrel, chopped
- ½ cup shallots, sliced thinly
- ¼ cup dry white wine
- 2 cups fish stock
- 2 tablespoons vermouth
- ½ cup fresh cream
- 4 salmon fillets
- Salt to taste
- 2 teaspoons olive oil

Instructions:

1. Add the water and sorrel in a blender.

2. Process until smooth.

3. Transfer to your bowl, cover and set aside.

4. In a pan over medium high heat, add the shallots, wine, fish stock and vermouth.

5. Bring to a boil. Reduce heat and simmer for 20 minutes.

6. Strain the sauce.

7. Put the sauce back to the pan and stir in the cream.

8. Transfer to your bowl, cover and set aside.

9. Next, sprinkle both sides of the salmon with the salt.

10. Pour the oil into a pan over medium heat.

11. Then, cook the salmon for 4 minutes per side.

12. Pour the sorrel and cream sauces over the salmon and serve.

Nutrients per Serving:

- *Calories 484*
- *Fat 33.4 g*
- *Saturated fat 11.9 g*
- *Carbohydrates 5.7 g*
- *Fiber 1.5 g*
- *Protein 33.7 g*
- *Cholesterol 104 mg*
- *Sugars 3 g*
- *Sodium 364 mg*
- *Potassium 870 mg*

Vegan Meatballs

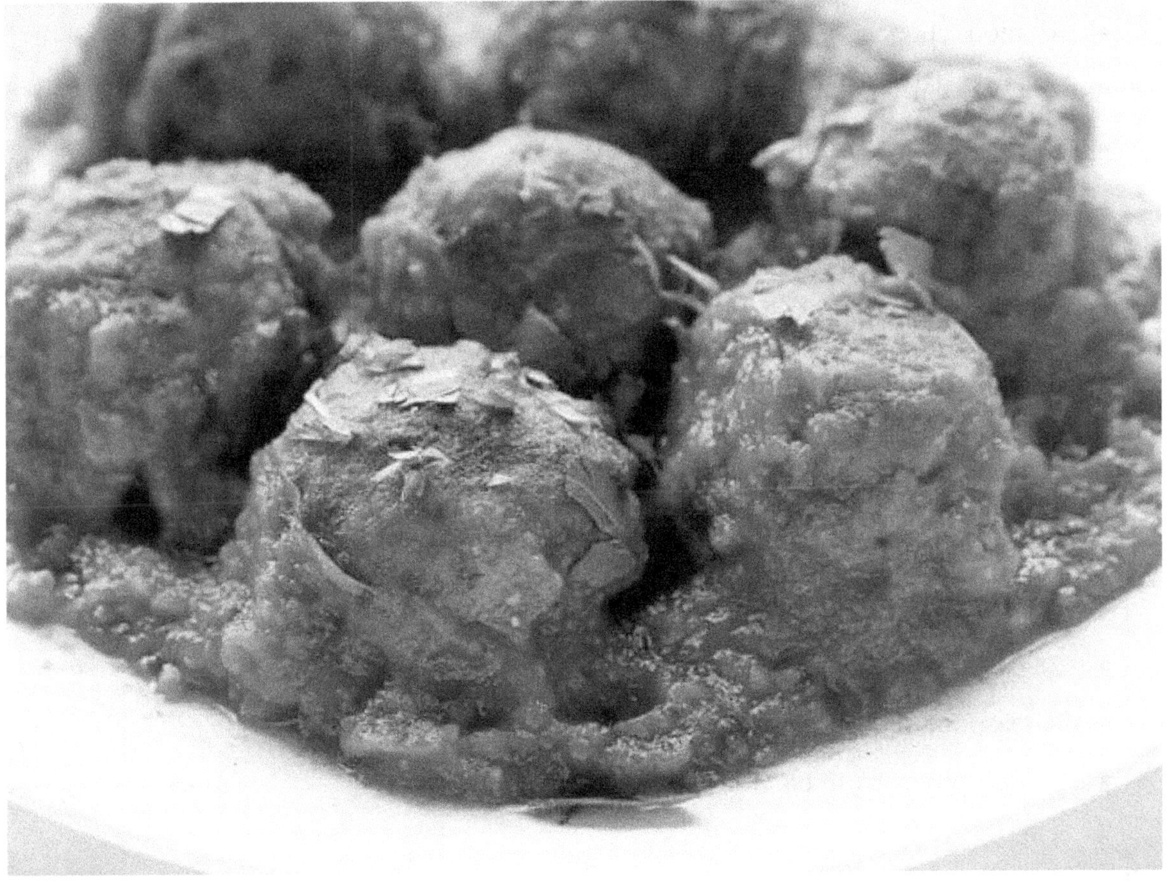

There's no need to adopt a vegan diet when you're pregnant. But you'd surely want to up your intake of fruits and vegetables. To make it easier for you to maintain a natural and plant-based diet, include recipes like this one in your weekly menu.

Serving Size: 6

Preparation Cooking Time: an hour and 10 minutes

Ingredients:

- Cooking spray
- 1 onion, chopped
- 2 cloves garlic, divided
- 8 oz. white mushrooms, sliced in half
- 2 ½ cups cauliflower florets
- 4 tablespoons olive oil, divided
- 1 ½ teaspoons Italian seasoning, divided
- Salt and pepper to taste
- 1 tablespoon tomato paste
- 1 cup canned chickpeas
- 1 tablespoon low-sodium soy sauce
- 2 cups quinoa, cooked
- 28 oz. canned crushed tomatoes
- ½ teaspoon red pepper flakes
- 2 tablespoons fresh basil leaves, chopped

Instructions:

1. Preheat your oven to 400 degrees F.

2. Spray your baking pan with oil.

3. Add the onion, 1 clove garlic, mushrooms and cauliflower in a food processor.

4. Pulse until chopped.

5. Pour half of the olive oil in a pan over medium heat.

6. Add the ground cauliflower mixture, half of the Italian seasoning, and the salt and pepper.

7. Stir and cook for 5 minutes.

8. Next, stir in the tomato paste. Cook for 1 more minute.

9. Transfer to a bowl. Let cool.

10. Puree the chickpeas in the food processor.

11. Add this to the bowl with the cauliflower mixture and mix with the soy sauce and quinoa.

12. Form into balls.

13. Add the meatballs to a baking pan.

14. Bake in the oven for 25 minutes.

15. Chop the remaining clove of garlic.

16. Then, add the remaining oil to a pan over medium heat.

17. Cook the garlic, and the rest of the ingredients.

18. Season with the salt and Italian seasoning.

19. Bring to a simmer for 5 minutes.

20. Pour the sauce over the meatballs.

21. Garnish with the basil leaves and serve.

Nutrients per Serving:

- *Calories 394*
- *Fat 17.1 g*
- *Saturated fat 2.4 g*
- *Carbohydrates 45.7 g*
- *Fiber 10.1 g*
- *Protein 12.7 g*
- *Cholesterol 3 mg*
- *Sugars 12 g*
- *Sodium 434 mg*
- *Potassium 1272 mg*

Crab Cakes

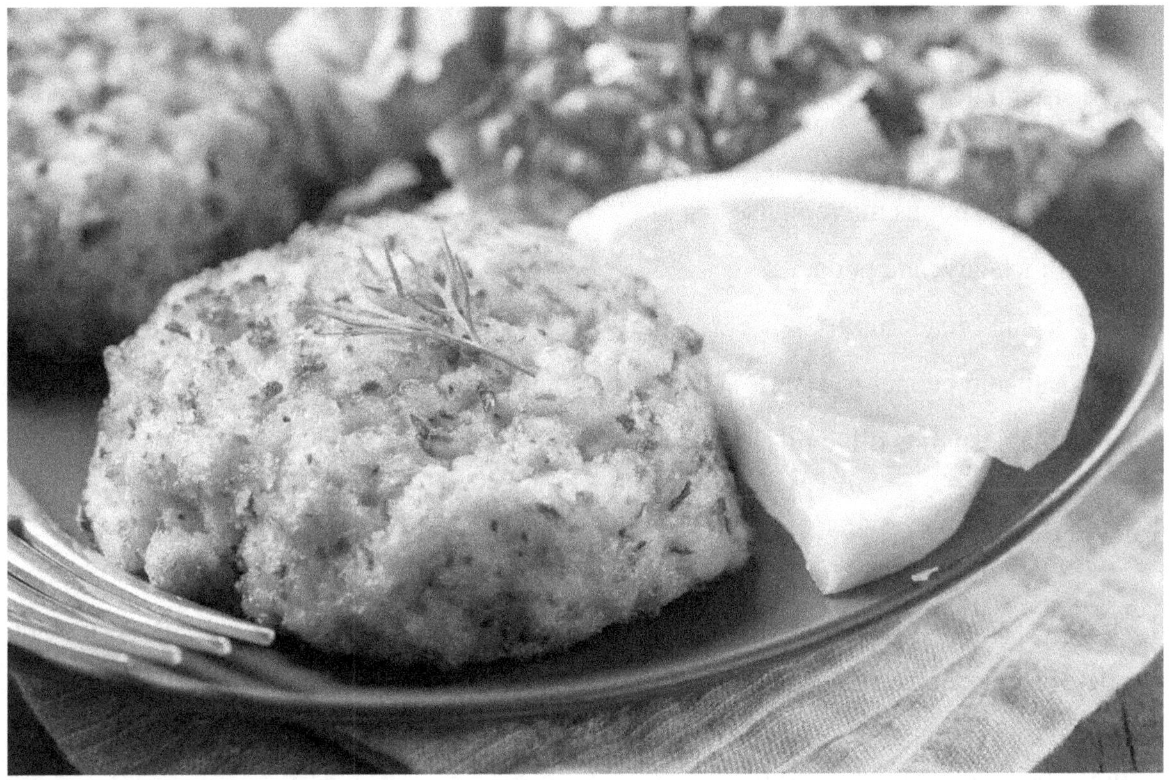

Get the golden crisp of these crab cakes without having to deep fry these in loads of oil.

Serving Size: 4

Preparation Cooking Time: 30 minutes

Ingredients:

- 12 oz. crabmeat
- ¼ cup scallions, chopped
- 1 egg, beaten
- 2 teaspoons Dijon mustard
- 2 tablespoons mayonnaise
- Pinch cayenne pepper
- ¾ cup breadcrumbs
- Salt and pepper to taste
- 2 tablespoons olive oil

Instructions:

1. In a bowl, combine the crabmeat, scallions, egg, mustard, mayonnaise, cayenne pepper, breadcrumbs, salt and pepper.

2. Form patties from the mixture.

3. Pour the oil into a pan over medium heat.

4. Cook the crab cakes for 4 minutes per side.

Nutrients per Serving:

- *Calories 265*
- *Fat 14.8 g*
- *Saturated fat 2.2 g*
- *Carbohydrates 11.2 g*
- *Fiber 1.7 g*
- *Protein 22 g*
- *Cholesterol 109 mg*
- *Sugars 1 g*
- *Sodium 486 mg*
- *Potassium 41 mg*

Taco Salad

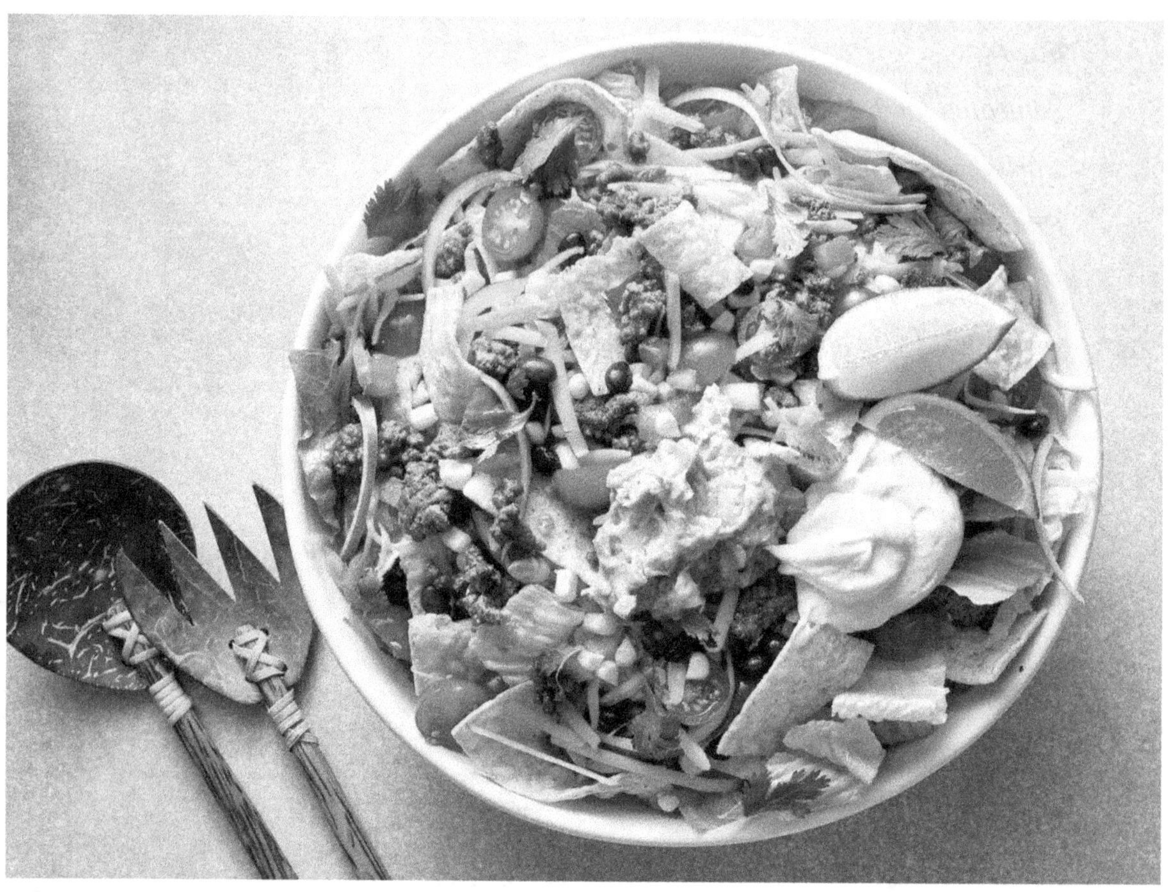

You love tacos but you don't like the greasy beef that comes with it. Don't fret. Here's a taco salad that you'll enjoy more. It supplies you with your much-needed protein, thanks to the black beans and tofu but packs in more nutrients than the usual recipe.

Serving Size: 2

Preparation Cooking Time: 15 minutes

Ingredients:

- 4 oz. tofu
- 3 cups Romaine lettuce, shredded
- ½ cup black beans, rinsed and drained
- ¾ cup tomatoes, chopped
- 8 tortilla chips
- ¼ cup low-fat cheddar cheese, shredded
- 1 tablespoon salsa
- 2 tablespoons light sour cream

Instructions:

1. Follow the package directions in preparing the tofu.

2. Place the Romaine lettuce in a salad bowl.

3. Sprinkle the tofu on top of the Romaine lettuce.

4. Sprinkle the rest of the ingredients on top except the last 2.

5. Serve with the salsa and sour cream.

Nutrients per Serving:

- *Calories 235*
- *Fat 7.6 g*
- *Saturated fat 3.6 g*
- *Carbohydrates 26.6 g*
- *Fiber 6.2 g*
- *Protein 17.4 g*
- *Cholesterol 36 mg*
- *Sugars 5 g*
- *Sodium 549 mg*
- *Potassium 544 mg*

Kale Dolmas

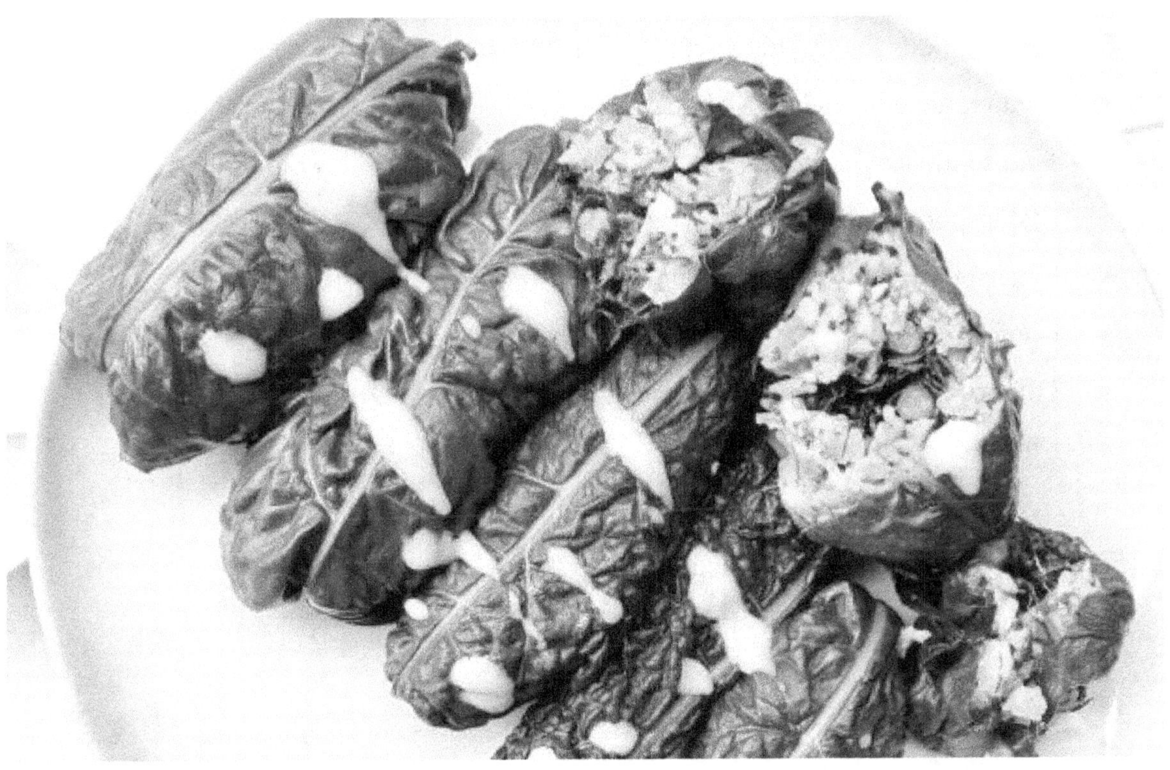

The popular Dolmas recipe wrapped with kale leaves—quick and easy meal for you to prepare without the fuss.

Serving Size: 4

Preparation Cooking Time: 45 minutes

Ingredients:

- 16 whole kale leaves
- 3 tablespoons lemon juice, freshly squeezed and divided
- ½ cup reduced-fat Greek yogurt
- 4 cups kale leaves, chopped
- 1 tablespoon olive oil
- 1 teaspoon freshly grated lemon zest
- 1 onion, chopped
- 3 cloves garlic, crushed and minced
- 1 lb. lean ground beef
- 2 cups brown rice, cooked
- ½ cup fresh parsley, chopped
- 2 tablespoons fresh dill, chopped
- Salt and pepper to taste

Instructions:

1. Fill a pot with water.

2. Bring to a boil.

3. Add the kale leaves and cook for 3 minutes.

4. Remove the kale leaves and drain on kitchen towel lined plates.

5. Drain the water from your pot and wipe it.

6. In a bowl, mix half of the lemon juice with the yogurt, salt and pepper. Set aside.

7. Pour the oil into a pan over medium heat.

8. Cook the chopped kale, onion and garlic for 1 minute.

9. Stir in the beef and cook for 4 minutes.

10. Add the rest of the ingredients along with the remaining lemon juice.

11. Season with the salt and pepper.

12. Cook for 2 minutes.

13. Place the whole kale leaves on a cutting board.

14. Add the beef mixture in the middle.

15. Fold the ends and roll into a cylinder.

16. Serve with the yogurt sauce.

Nutrients per Serving:

- *Calories 471*
- *Fat 16.5 g*
- *Saturated fat 5.6 g*
- *Carbohydrates 48.6 g*
- *Fiber 6.4 g*
- *Protein 34.5 g*
- *Cholesterol 77 mg*
- *Sugars 3 g*
- *Sodium 748 mg*
- *Potassium 607 mg*

Egg Cheese

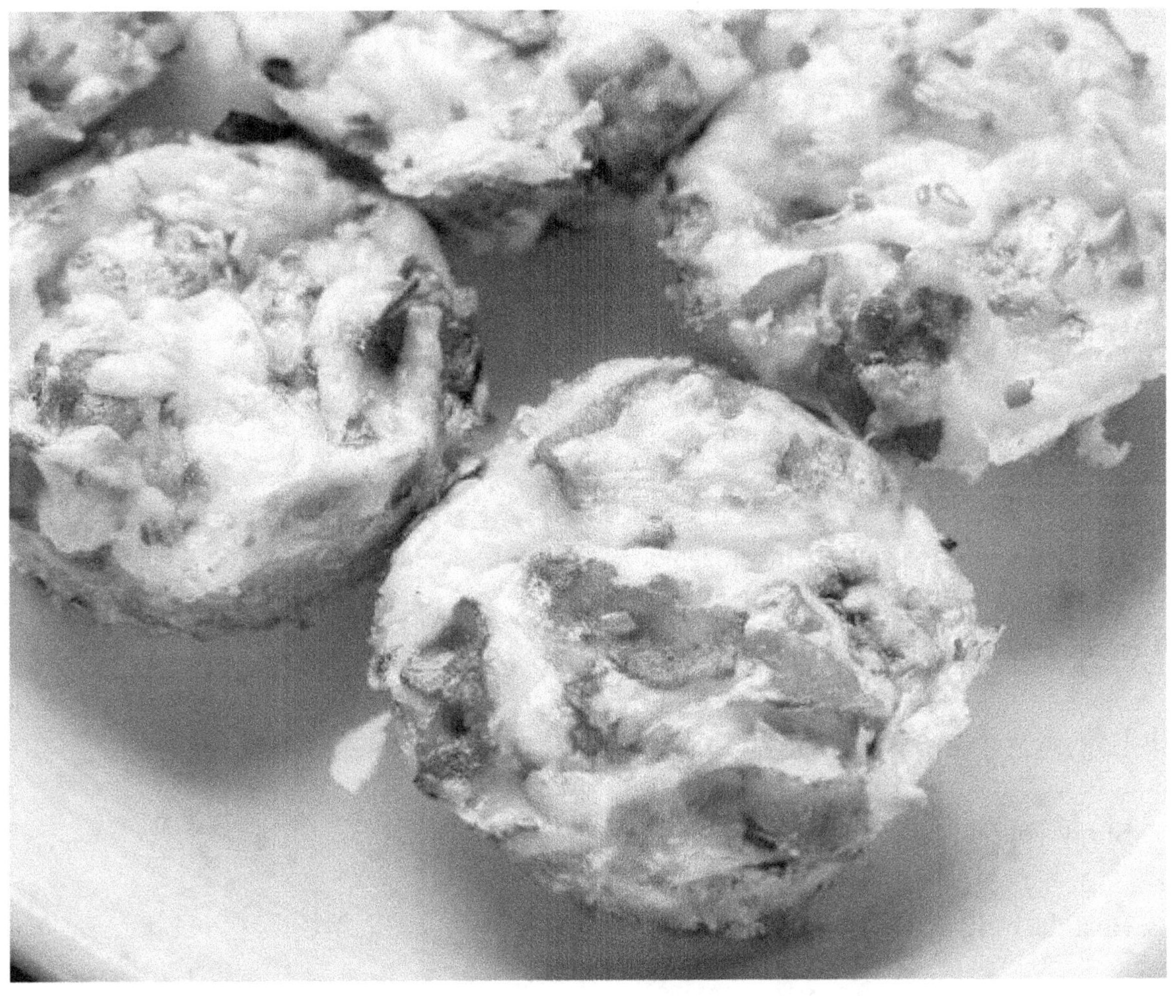

Make egg and cheese sandwiches the unique way using this simple and easy to follow recipe.

Serving Size: 12

Preparation Cooking Time: 50 minutes

Ingredients:

- ¼ cup low-fat milk
- 18 eggs, beaten
- 1 teaspoon onion powder
- ½ teaspoon ground cumin
- 1 tablespoon chili powder
- Salt and pepper to taste
- 10 oz. spinach, chopped
- ¾ cup red bell pepper, chopped
- 1 cup cheddar cheese, shredded
- 4 slices bacon, cooked and chopped
- 12 whole-wheat muffins, toasted

Instructions:

1. Preheat your oven to 300 degrees F.

2. Spray your baking pan with oil.

3. Beat the milk and eggs in a bowl.

4. Stir in the onion powder, cumin, chili powder, salt and pepper.

5. Pour the mixture into a baking pan.

6. Sprinkle the cheese, spinach, bacon and red bell pepper on top.

7. Bake in the oven for 25 minutes.

8. Slice into 12 squares and place the slices on top of the muffins.

Nutrients per Serving:

- *Calories 309*
- *Fat 13.1 g*
- *Saturated fat 4.8 g*
- *Carbohydrates 30 g*
- *Fiber 5.6 g*
- *Protein 19.6 g*
- *Cholesterol 292 mg*
- *Sugars 7 g*
- *Sodium 688 mg*
- *Potassium 391 mg*

Turkey Burger with Sweet Potato Fries

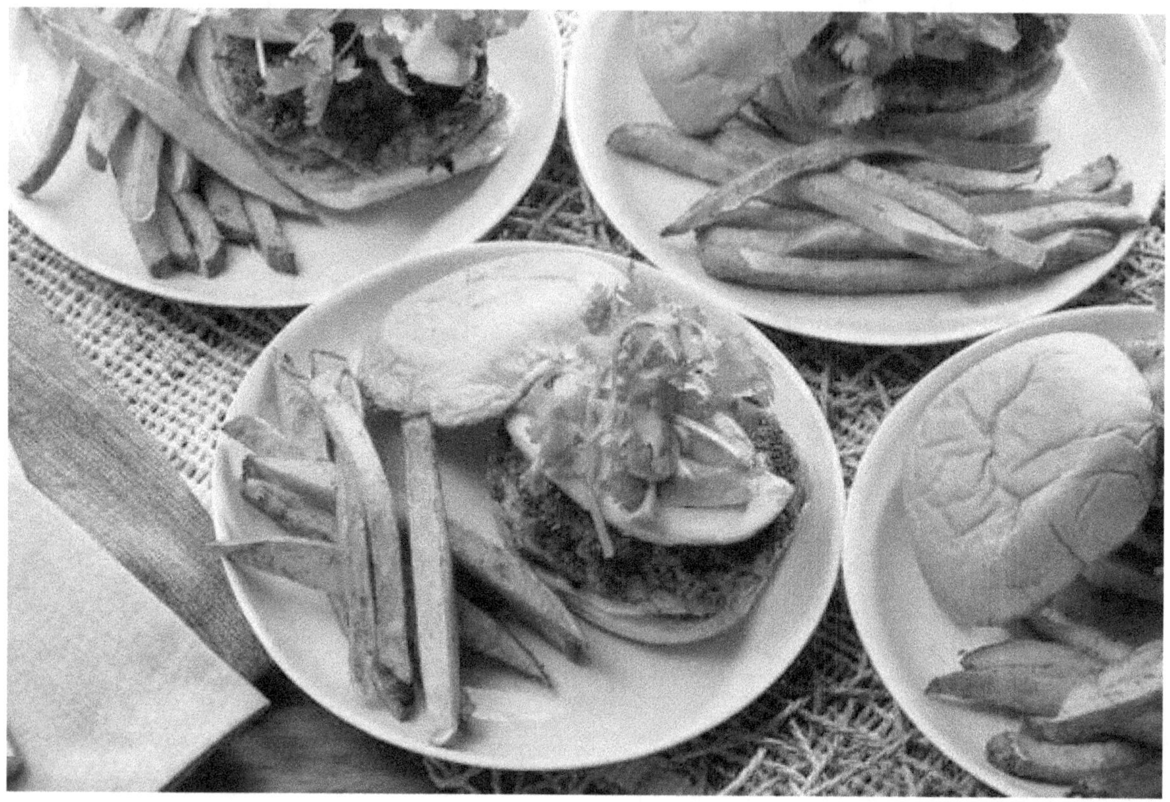

Here's another way to enjoy your burger without loading up too much fat and calories—make your patty from ground turkey. Not only that, you should also top it with thick slices of avocado and pair it up with sweet potato fries.

Serving Size: 2

Preparation Cooking Time: 30 minutes

Ingredients:

- 1 sweet potato, slices into strips
- 2 teaspoons vegetable oil
- Salt to taste

Burgers

- 8 oz. lean ground turkey
- ¼ cup cheddar cheese, shredded
- 2 teaspoons Worcestershire sauce
- ½ teaspoon garlic powder
- Salt and pepper to taste
- 2 teaspoons vegetable oil
- 2 slices sweet onion
- 2 slices tomato
- ½ avocado, sliced thickly
- 5 lettuce leaves

Instructions:

1. Preheat your oven to 425 degrees F.

2. Toss the sweet potato fries in oil and season with the salt.

3. Bake in the oven for 10 minutes.

4. Flip and bake for another 10 minutes.

5. Set aside.

6. Next, in a bowl, mix all the ingredients for the burger.

7. Form into patties.

8. Coat the pan with oil.

9. Then, cook the patties for 2 minutes per side.

10. Cover the pan and cook for 2 more minutes.

11. Top the burgers with the slices of onion, tomato and avocado.

12. Cover with the lettuce leaves.

13. Serve with the sweet potato fries.

Nutrients per Serving:

- *Calories 463*
- *Fat 23.1 g*
- *Saturated fat 6.3 g*
- *Carbohydrates 33.5 g*
- *Fiber 7.9 g*
- *Protein 35.4 g*
- *Cholesterol 58 mg*
- *Sugars 10 g*
- *Sodium 690 mg*
- *Potassium 777 mg*

Pasta Salad

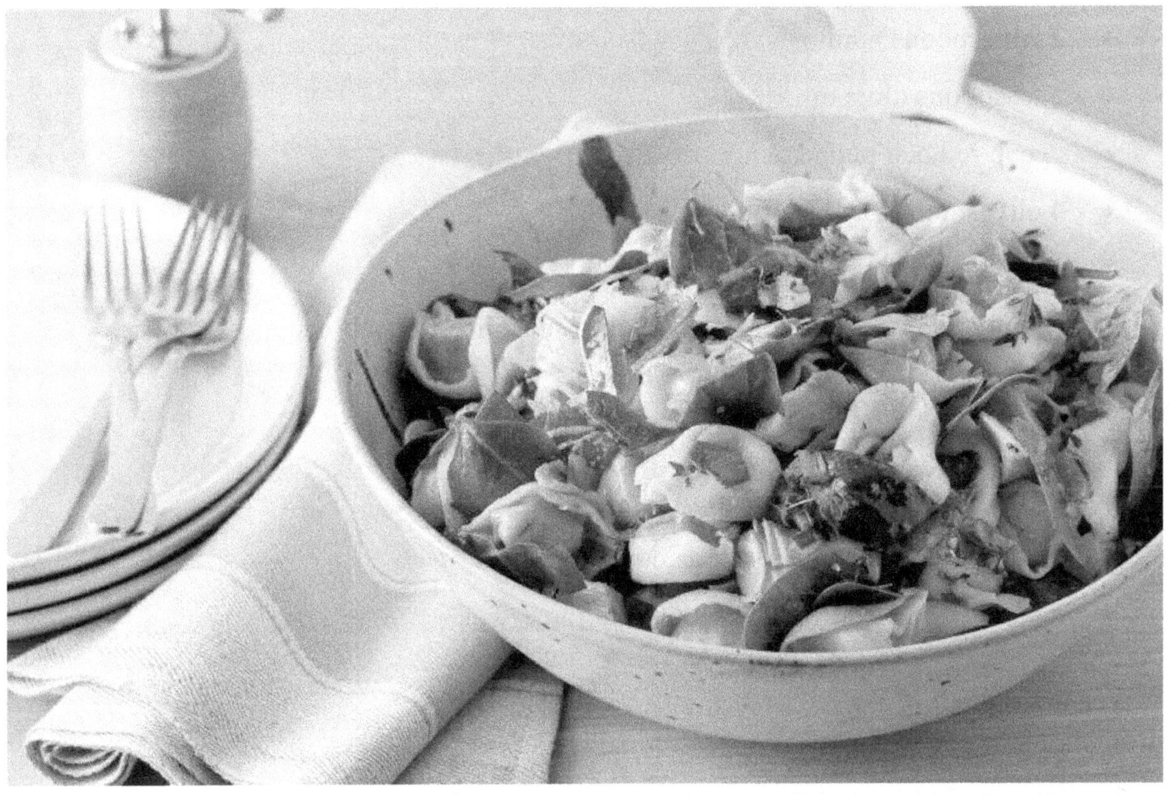

Here's a unique take on your favorite pasta salad—instead of tossing it in mayo sauce, you make use of hummus to infuse it with exciting Mediterranean flavors.

Serving Size: 1

Preparation Cooking Time: 20 minutes

Ingredients:

- 1 tablespoon water
- 2 tablespoons hummus
- 2 teaspoons olive oil
- ½ cup red bell pepper, chopped
- 4 olives, pitted and chopped
- 1 cup kale, chopped
- ½ cup artichoke hearts, rinsed, drained and sliced in half
- 3 oz. canned tuna flakes, drained
- ½ cup whole-wheat farfalle, cooked
- 1 tablespoon feta cheese, crumbled
- 1 tablespoon walnuts, toasted and chopped
- 1 tablespoon freshly squeezed lemon juice

Instructions:

1. Combine the water and hummus in a bowl.

2. Pour the oil into a pan over medium heat.

3. Cook the bell pepper for 1 minute.

4. Stir in the olives, kale and artichokes.

5. Add the tuna and toss to combine.

6. Cook for 1 minute.

7. Remove from heat.

8. Add the pasta and the hummus sauce.

9. Sprinkle the walnuts and feta on top.

10. Drizzle with the lemon juice before serving.

Nutrients per Serving:

- *Calories 506*
- *Fat 24.5 g*
- *Saturated fat 4 g*
- *Carbohydrates 38.3 g*
- *Fiber 7 g*
- *Protein 33.4 g*
- *Cholesterol 34 mg*
- *Sugars 3 g*
- *Sodium 747 mg*
- *Potassium 540 mg*

Chicken Burrito

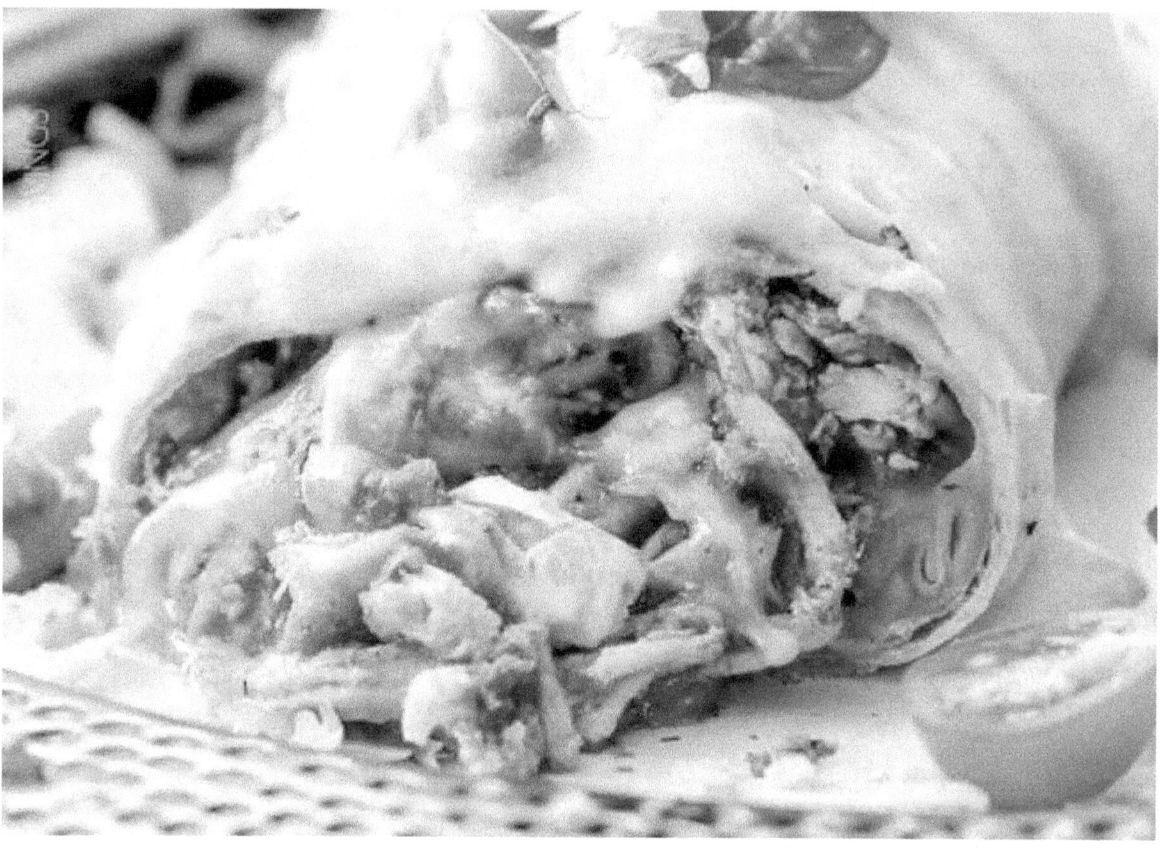

Have leftover chicken from last night's dinner? Use it to stuff your healthy burrito. You can even freeze this for later use.

Serving Size: 4

Preparation Cooking Time: 30 minutes

Ingredients:

- 2 teaspoons avocado oil
- ½ cup onion, chopped
- 1 teaspoons garlic, crushed and minced
- 1 tablespoons chipotle pepper in adobo sauce, minced
- 15 oz. canned reduced-sodium black beans, rinsed and drained
- ½ cup water
- 2 cups kale, chopped
- 2 cups chicken, cooked and shredded
- 2 tablespoons cilantro, chopped
- 1 cup low-fat cheddar cheese
- 1 tablespoon freshly squeezed lime juice
- ½ teaspoon freshly grated lime zest
- Salt to taste
- 4 whole-wheat tortillas

Instructions:

1. Pour the oil into a pan over medium heat.

2. Cook the onion and garlic for 2 minutes.

3. Stir in the chipotle pepper, black beans and water.

4. Simmer for 5 minutes.

5. Mash the beans gently with a spatula.

6. Stir in the kale and chicken.

7. Cook for 2 minutes.

8. Remove from the stove.

9. Add the cilantro, cheese, lime juice, lime zest and salt.

10. Mix well.

11. Spread the filling on top of the tortillas.

12. Roll each one tightly.

Nutrients per Serving:

- *Calories 375*
- *Fat 8.7 g*
- *Saturated fat 2.4 g*
- *Carbohydrates 44.3 g*
- *Fiber 0.7 g*
- *Protein 26.5 g*
- *Cholesterol 30 mg*
- *Sugars 4 g*
- *Sodium 854 mg*
- *Potassium 417 mg*

Garlic Chicken

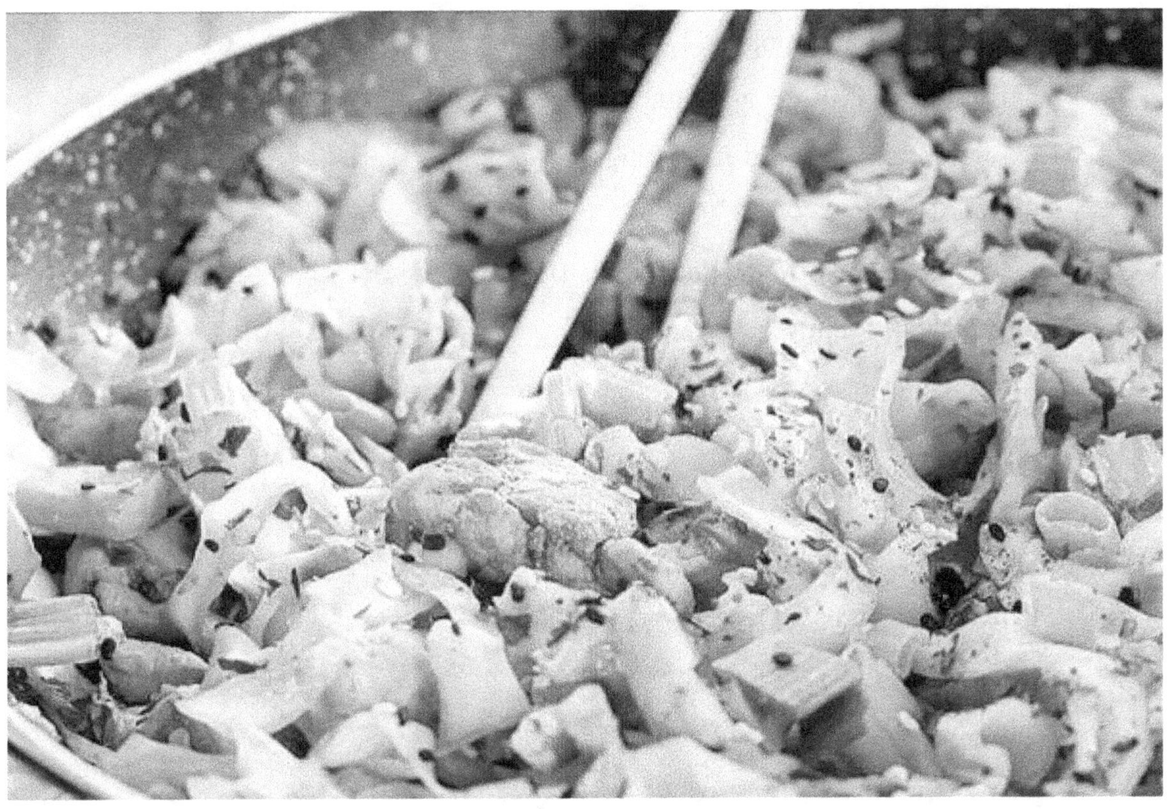

Stir-fries are some of the simplest and quickest dishes you can prepare for yourself and your family. In this recipe, we cook the chicken in garlic, and sauté it with colorful vegetables for more nutrients and extra crunch.

Serving Size: 4

Preparation Cooking Time: 20 minutes

Ingredients:

- 2 tablespoons peanut oil
- 1 cup green onions, chopped
- 6 cloves garlic, crushed and minced
- 1 teaspoon freshly grated fresh ginger
- Salt to taste
- 1 lb. chicken breast fillet, sliced into strips
- 2 onions, sliced thinly
- 1 red bell pepper, sliced into the thin strips
- 2 cups sugar snap peas
- 1 cup cabbage, sliced
- 1 cup reduced-sodium chicken broth, divided
- 2 tablespoons cornstarch
- 2 tablespoons reduced-sodium soy sauce
- 2 tablespoons white sugar

Instructions:

1. Add the peanut oil to a pan over medium high heat.

2. Once hot, add the green onions, garlic and ginger.

3. Season with the salt.

4. Stir in the chicken.

5. Cook for 3 minutes, stirring frequently.

6. Stir in the onions, red bell pepper, cabbage and sugar snap peas.

7. Pour in half of the broth.

8. Cover the pan.

9. In a bowl, mix the remaining broth with the cornstarch, soy sauce and sugar.

10. Pour this mixture into the pan and simmer until thickened.

Nutrients per Serving:

- *Calories 337*
- *Fat 8.6 g*
- *Saturated fat 1.6 g*
- *Carbohydrates 32.3 g*
- *Fiber 5.9 g*
- *Protein 31.7 g*
- *Cholesterol 67 mg*
- *Sugars 12 g*
- *Sodium 1364 mg*
- *Potassium 664 mg*

Lemon Pepper Fish

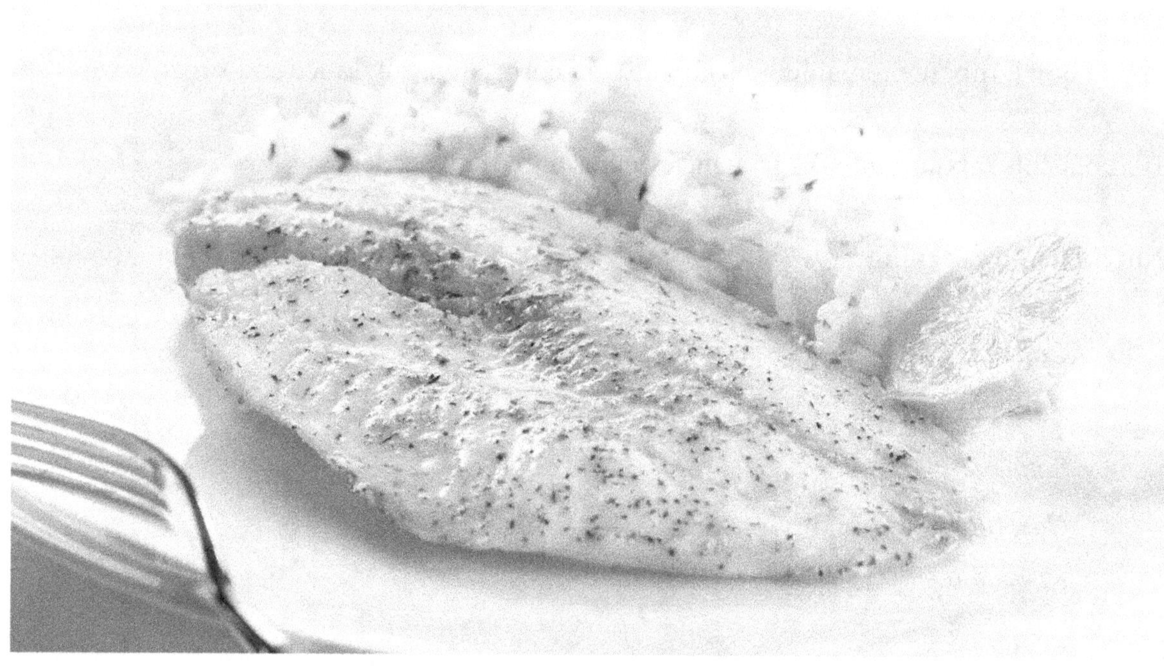

Fish fillet seasoned with lemon pepper and made even more delicious with tomatoes and couscous.

Serving Size: 4

Preparation Cooking Time: 30 minutes

Ingredients:

- 2 tablespoons olive oil
- 2 tablespoons butter
- 4 white fish or salmon fillets
- Salt to taste
- 1 tablespoon lemon pepper
- 1 teaspoon garlic, crushed and minced
- ¼ cup water
- 1 cup fresh cilantro, chopped
- 1 cup fresh tomatoes, chopped
- 2 cups hot water
- 1 cup uncooked couscous

Instructions:

1. Pour the olive oil and butter in a pan over medium heat.

2. Season both sides of the fish with salt, lemon pepper and garlic.

3. Add the fish in the pan along with the water, cilantro and tomatoes.

4. Cover the pan and cook for 15 minutes.

5. Pour the hot water into a bowl.

6. Add the couscous.

7. Cover and wait for 5 minutes.

8. Serve the salmon with the couscous and sauce from the pan.

Nutrients per Serving:

- *Calories 498*
- *Fat 23.5 g*
- *Saturated fat 7 g*
- *Carbohydrates 36.2 g*
- *Fiber 3.1 g*
- *Protein 31.6 g*
- *Cholesterol 89 mg*
- *Sugars 1 g*
- *Sodium 1039 mg*
- *Potassium 701 mg*

Cucumber Avocado Salad

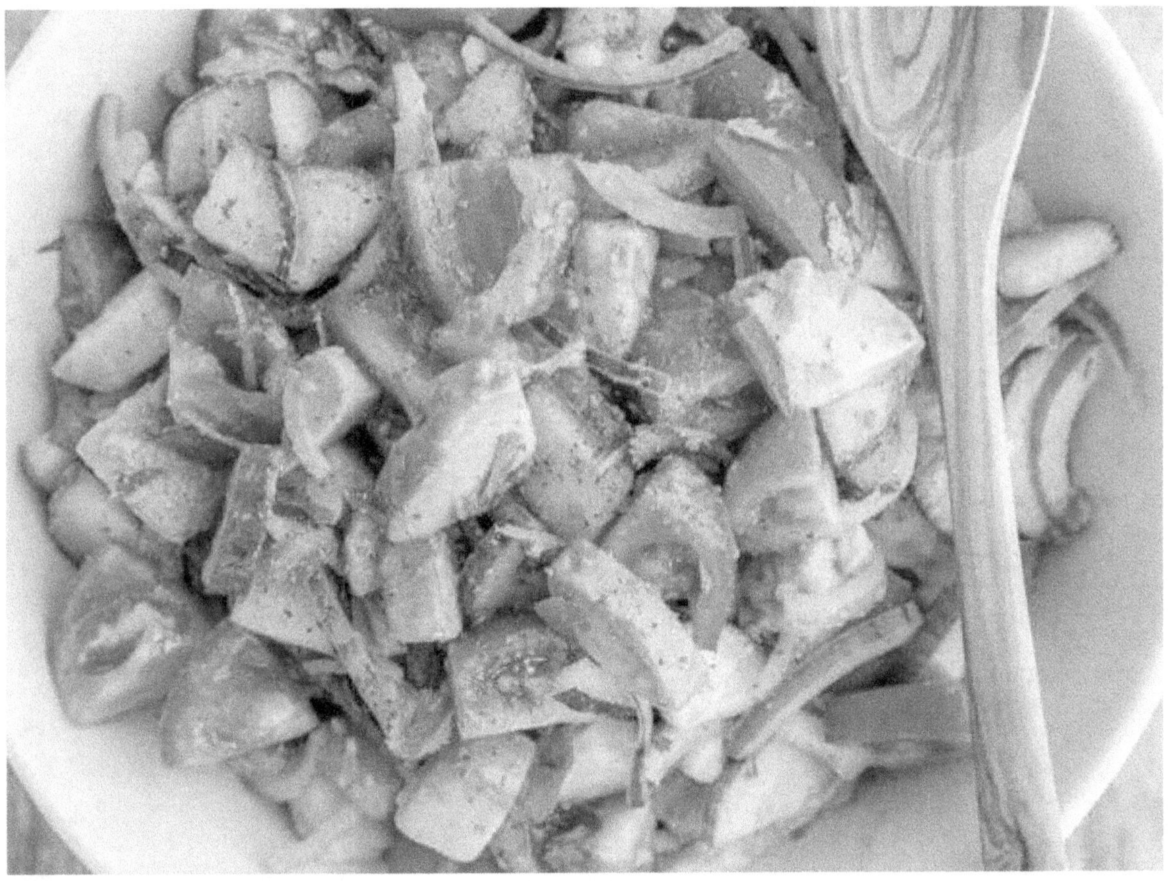

This dish is simple to make but gives you lots of bright colors and delicious flavors. The spiralized veggies are topped with creamy avocado dressing.

Serving Size: 4

Preparation Cooking Time: 50 minutes

Ingredients:

- 1 onion, sliced into rings
- 2 bell peppers, sliced into strips
- 1 jicama, spiralized
- 1 zucchini, spiralized
- 1 jalapeno pepper, spiralized
- 1 lime, juiced
- 1 tablespoon avocado oil
- 2 ripe avocados, mashed
- Garlic salt to taste
- 4 tostada shells
- 10 cherry tomatoes, sliced in half
- 1 lime, sliced into wedges
- ¼ cup cilantro, chopped

Instructions:

1. Toss the onion, bell pepper, cucumber and jicama in a bowl.

2. In another bowl, mix the avocado oil and lime juice.

3. Refrigerate for 20 minutes.

4. Sprinkle the mashed avocado with the garlic salt.

5. Spread the tostada shells with the avocado mixture.

6. Top with the tomatoes and jicama mix.

7. Serve with the lime wedges and cilantro.

Nutrients per Serving:

- *Calories 175*
- *Fat 6.2 g*
- *Saturated fat 1 g*
- *Carbohydrates 28.2 g*
- *Fiber 9.8 g*
- *Protein 3.1 g*
- *Cholesterol 0 mg*
- *Sugars 5 g*
- *Sodium 5 mg*
- *Potassium 488 mg*

Squash Soup

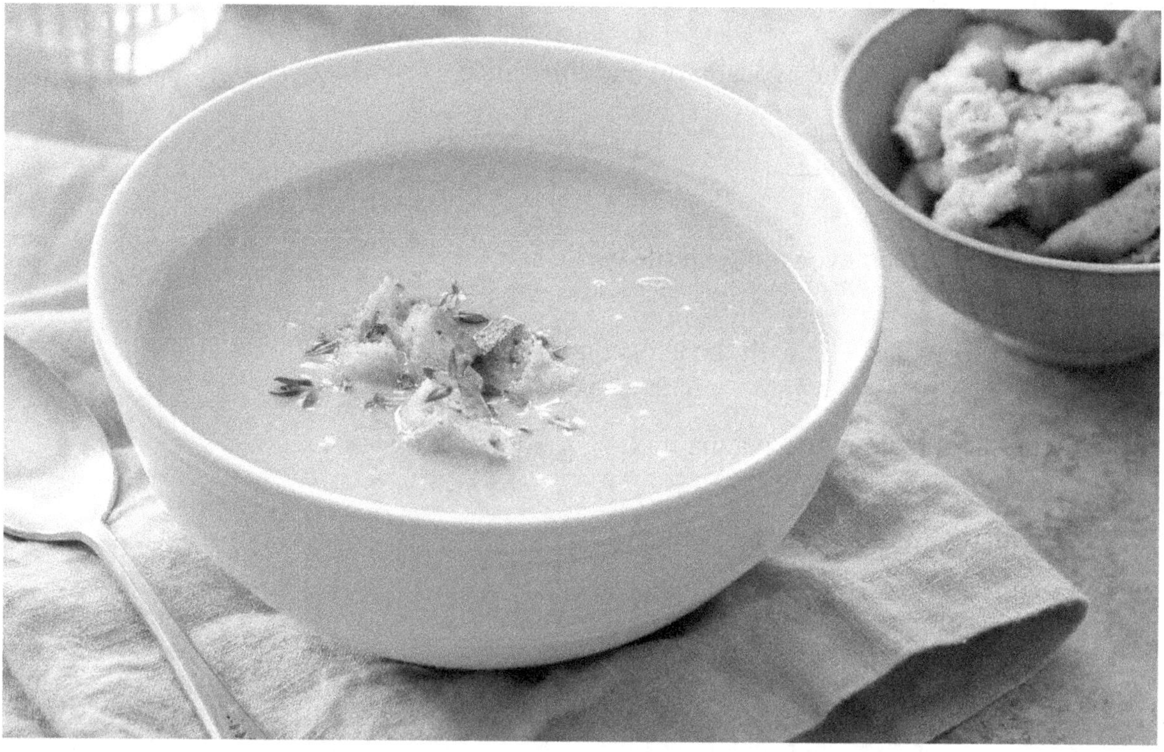

This comforting butternut squash soup is best served with curried almonds or toasted pumpkin seeds.

Serving Size: 4

Preparation Cooking Time: 2 hours

Ingredients:

- 1 butternut squash, sliced into cubes
- 1 tablespoon olive oil
- 1 onion, chopped
- 1 shallot, minced
- 2 tablespoons curry powder
- 1 teaspoon ground turmeric
- 1 apple, sliced into small pieces
- 1 slice ginger, minced
- Water
- 14 oz. coconut milk
- Salt to taste

Instructions:

1. Preheat your oven to 350 degrees F.

2. Bake for 45 minutes.

3. Pour the oil into a pan over medium heat.

4. Cook the onion and shallot for 10 minutes.

5. Stir in the turmeric and curry powder.

6. Cook for 2 minutes.

7. Add the apple, ginger and squash into the pan.

8. Cover with the water.

9. Bring to a boil.

10. Reduce heat and simmer for 15 minutes.

11. Transfer the mixture to a blender.

12. Process until smooth.

13. Combine the salt and coconut milk in a pan.

14. Simmer for 3 minutes.

15. Add to the soup and heat through for 1 minute before serving.

Nutrients per Serving:

- *Calories 388*
- *Fat 25.1 g*
- *Saturated fat 19 g*
- *Carbohydrates 44.3 g*
- *Fiber 8.8 g*
- *Protein 5.7 g*
- *Cholesterol 0 mg*
- *Sugars 11 g*
- *Sodium 68 mg*
- *Potassium 1299 mg*

Mediterranean Chicken

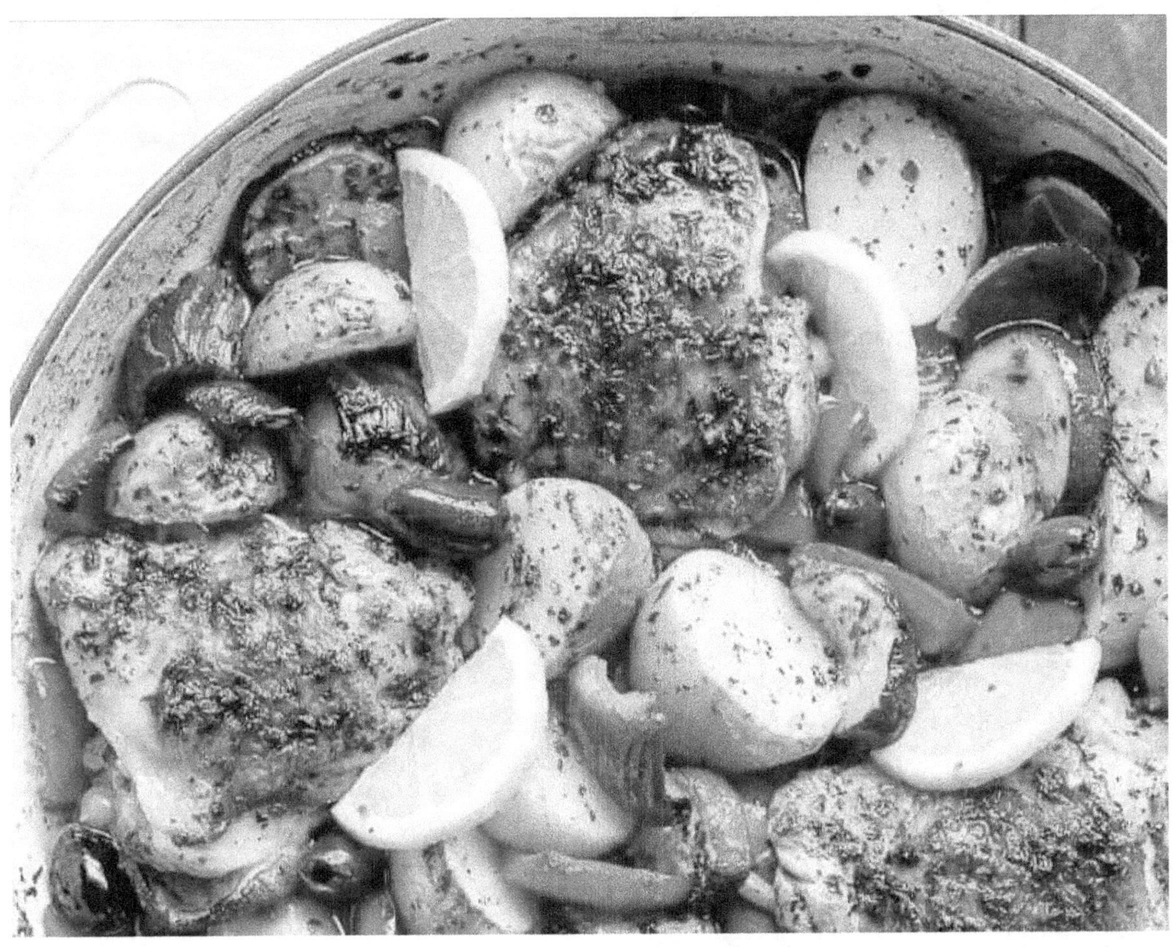

Sauté chicken and simmer it in tomato sauce made more flavorful with garlic, herbs, olives and white wine.

Serving Size: 6

Preparation Cooking Time: 30 minutes

Ingredients:

- 2 teaspoons olive oil
- 2 tablespoons white wine
- 6 chicken breast fillet
- 3 cloves garlic, crushed and minced
- ½ cup onion, diced
- 3 cups tomatoes, diced
- ½ cup white wine
- 1 tablespoon fresh basil, chopped
- 2 teaspoons thyme leaves, chopped
- ½ cup olives, pitted
- ¼ cup fresh parsley, chopped
- Salt and pepper to taste

Instructions:

1. Pour the oil and wine in a pan over medium heat.

2. Add the chicken and cook for 5 minutes per side.

3. Transfer to a plate and set aside.

4. Cook the garlic in the drippings for 30 seconds.

5. Add the onion and cook for 3 minutes.

6. Stir in the tomatoes.

7. Bring to a boil.

8. Reduce heat.

9. Add the white wine into the pan.

10. Cook for 10 minutes.

11. Stir in the herbs and cook for 5 minutes.

12. Put the chicken back to the pan.

13. Cook the chicken for 10 minutes per side.

14. Stir in the parsley and olives and cook for 1 minute.

15. Season with the salt and pepper.

Nutrients per Serving:

- *Calories 222*
- *Fat 6.2 g*
- *Saturated fat 1 g*
- *Carbohydrates 7.2 g*
- *Fiber 1.6 g*
- *Protein 28.6 g*
- *Cholesterol 68 mg*
- *Sugars 3 g*
- *Sodium 268 mg*
- *Potassium 575 mg*

Vermicelli Noodles

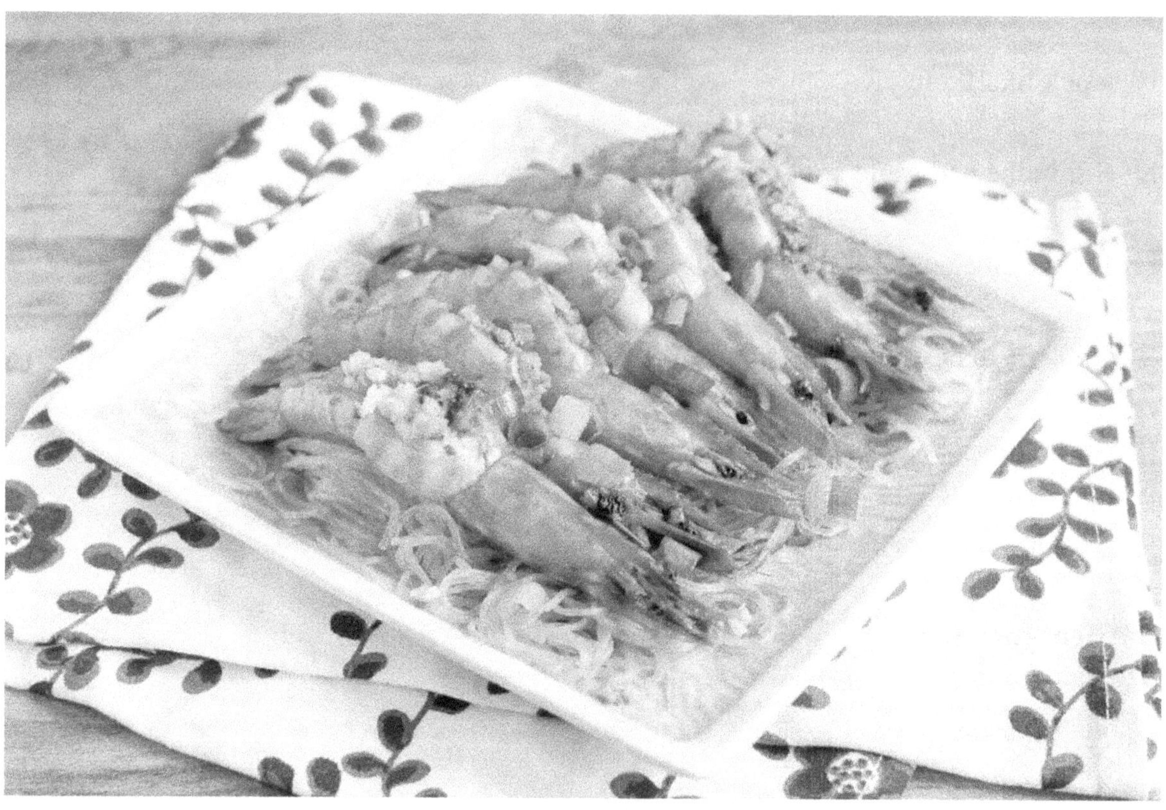

This one is a popular Vietnamese dish that would fill you up and delight you with loads of flavors. It combines rice noodles, cucumber, grilled shrimp, herbs, bean sprouts and sweet savory sauce.

Serving Size: 2

Preparation Cooking Time: 1 hour

Ingredients:

- 1 clove garlic, crushed and minced
- ¼ cup fish sauce
- ¼ cup white vinegar
- 2 tablespoons freshly squeezed lime juice
- ¼ teaspoon red pepper flakes
- 2 tablespoons white sugar
- ½ teaspoon vegetable oil
- 2 tablespoons shallots, chopped
- 8 shrimp
- 8 oz. rice vermicelli noodles
- 1 cup bean sprouts
- 1 cup lettuce, chopped
- ¼ cup pickled carrots, chopped
- 1 zucchini, sliced into thin sticks
- 3 tablespoons cilantro, chopped
- ¼ cup diakon radish, chopped
- 3 tablespoons Thai basil, chopped
- ¼ cup peanuts, crushed
- 3 tablespoons fresh mint, chopped

Instructions:

1. Combine the garlic, fish sauce, vinegar, lime juice, red pepper flakes and sugar in a bowl. Set aside.

2. Pour the oil into a pan over medium heat.

3. Cook the shallots for 8 minutes.

4. Preheat your grill.

5. Thread the shrimp into the skewers.

6. Grill for 2 minutes per side. Set aside.

7. Boil a pot of water.

8. Cook the noodles for 12 minutes.

9. Drain and rinse under cool running water.

10. Stir to separate the rice noodles

11. Place the noodles in serving bowls.

12. Top with the remaining ingredients and grilled shrimp.

13. Pour the sauce into the bowl. Serve.

Nutrients per Serving:

- *Calories 659*
- *Fat 12.8 g*
- *Saturated fat 2 g*
- *Carbohydrates 112 g*
- *Fiber 8.6 g*
- *Protein 26.2 g*
- *Cholesterol 36 mg*
- *Sugars 19 g*
- *Sodium 2565 mg*
- *Potassium 756 mg*

Fiesta Salad

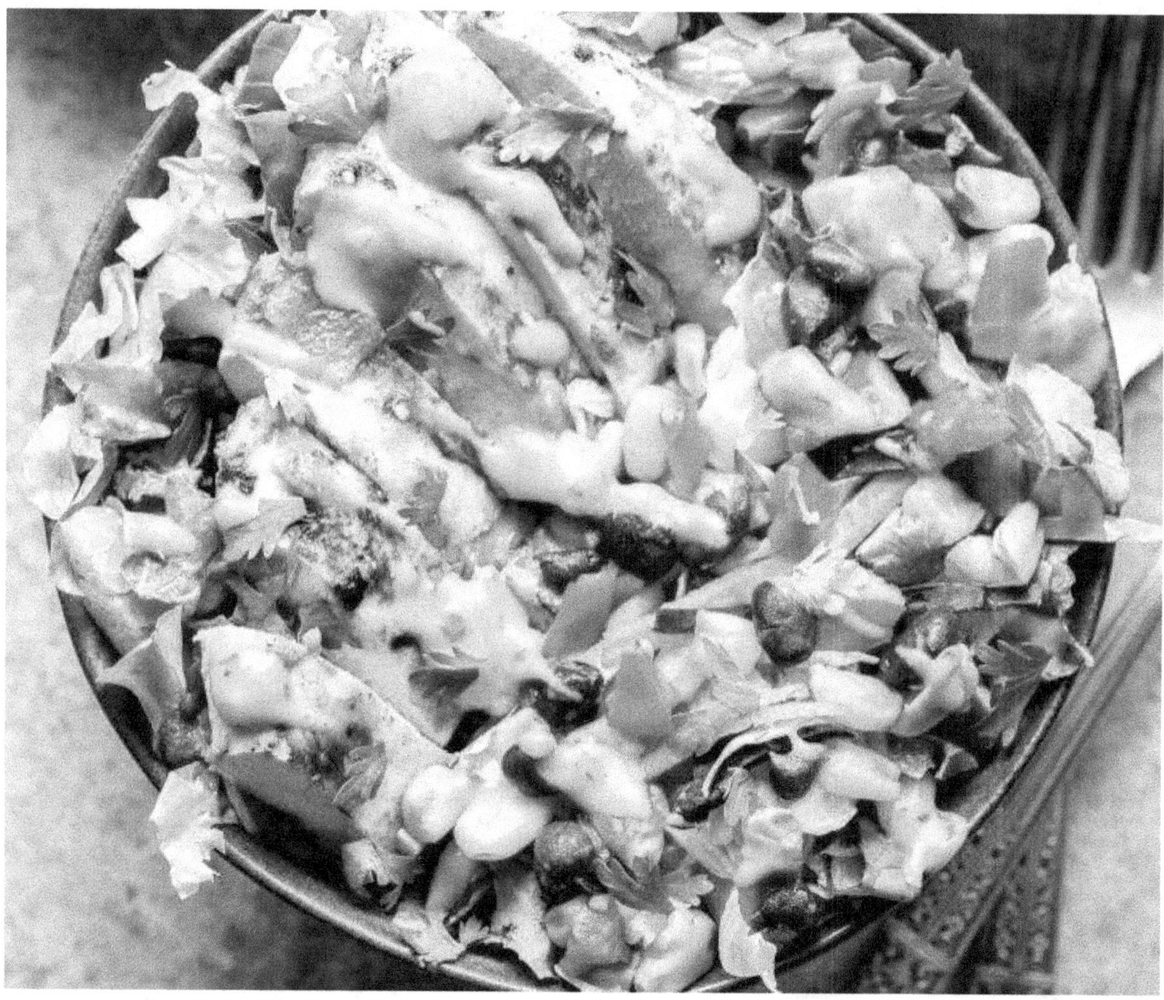

Here's something to fill you up but will not wreak havoc with your health—fiesta salad loaded with chicken, vegetables, shredded cheddar cheese and crumbled tortilla chips.

Serving Size: 4

Preparation Cooking Time: 40 minutes

Ingredients:

- 2 chicken breast fillet, sliced into strips
- 1 packet fajita seasoning, divided
- 1 tablespoon vegetable oil
- 11 oz. corn kernels
- 15 oz. black beans, rinsed and drained
- ½ cup salsa
- 10 oz. mixed salad greens
- 1 tomato, sliced into wedges
- 1 onion, chopped

Instructions:

1. Season the chicken with half of the fajita seasoning.

2. Pour the oil into a pan over medium heat.

3. Cook the chicken for 16 minutes, flipping once.

4. In a pan over medium heat, combine the corn, beans and salsa.

5. Season with the remaining fajita powder.

6. Stir well.

7. Toss the leafy greens, tomato and onion.

8. Top with the chicken and the corn mixture.

Nutrients per Serving:

- *Calories 311*
- *Fat 6.4 g*
- *Saturated fat 1.1 g*
- *Carbohydrates 42.2 g*
- *Fiber 10.5 g*
- *Protein 23 g*
- *Cholesterol 36 mg*
- *Sugars 7 g*
- *Sodium 1606 mg*
- *Potassium 540 mg*

Grilled Salmon with Blueberry Topping

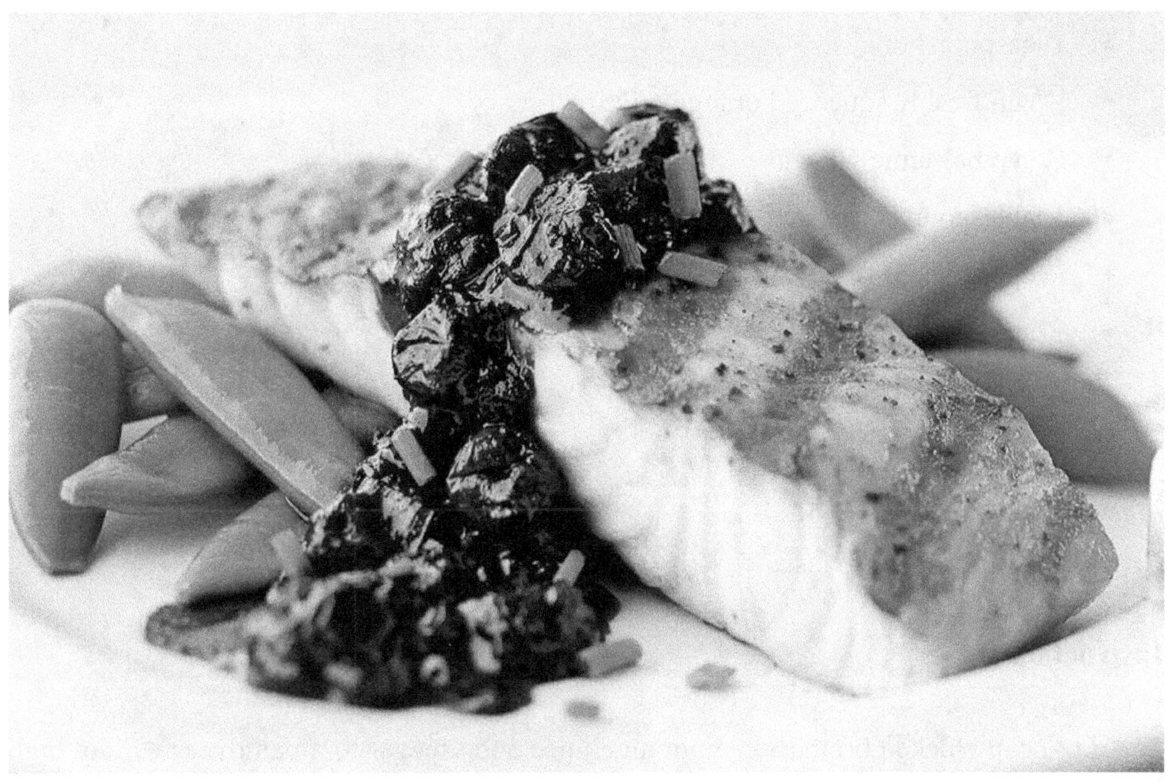

You probably couldn't imagine pairing grilled salmon with blueberries. In this recipe, we won't just pair the two, we'll pour the salmon steak with blueberry sauce to create an incredible fish you'd find hard not to crave for.

Serving Size: 4

Preparation Cooking Time: 25 minutes

Ingredients:

- ¾ cup chicken broth, divided
- 1 teaspoon honey
- ¼ cup freshly squeezed orange juice
- ¼ cup balsamic vinegar
- 1 tablespoon cornstarch
- ¼ cup chicken stock
- 1 cup fresh blueberries
- 2 teaspoons fresh chives, chopped
- 4 salmon fillets
- 2 tablespoons olive oil
- Salt and pepper to taste

Instructions:

1. Add ½ cup chicken broth, honey, orange juice and vinegar to a pan over medium high heat.

2. Bring to a boil.

3. Reduce heat.

4. Add ¼ cup chicken broth to a bowl.

5. Stir in the cornstarch until dissolved.

6. Pour the mixture into the pan.

7. Cook for 2 minutes.

8. Add the chives and blueberries.

9. Reduce heat to low. Cook for 2 minutes.

10. Coat the salmon with the oil.

11. Next, sprinkle both sides with the salt and pepper.

12. Grill the fish for 3 minutes per side.

13. Pour the blueberry sauce on top.

Nutrients per Serving:

- *Calories 383*
- *Fat 23.2 g*
- *Saturated fat 4 g*
- *Carbohydrates 12.8 g*
- *Fiber 0.9 g*
- *Protein 29.6 g*
- *Cholesterol 83 mg*
- *Sugars 9 g*
- *Sodium 265 mg*
- *Potassium 577 mg*

Zucchini Salad

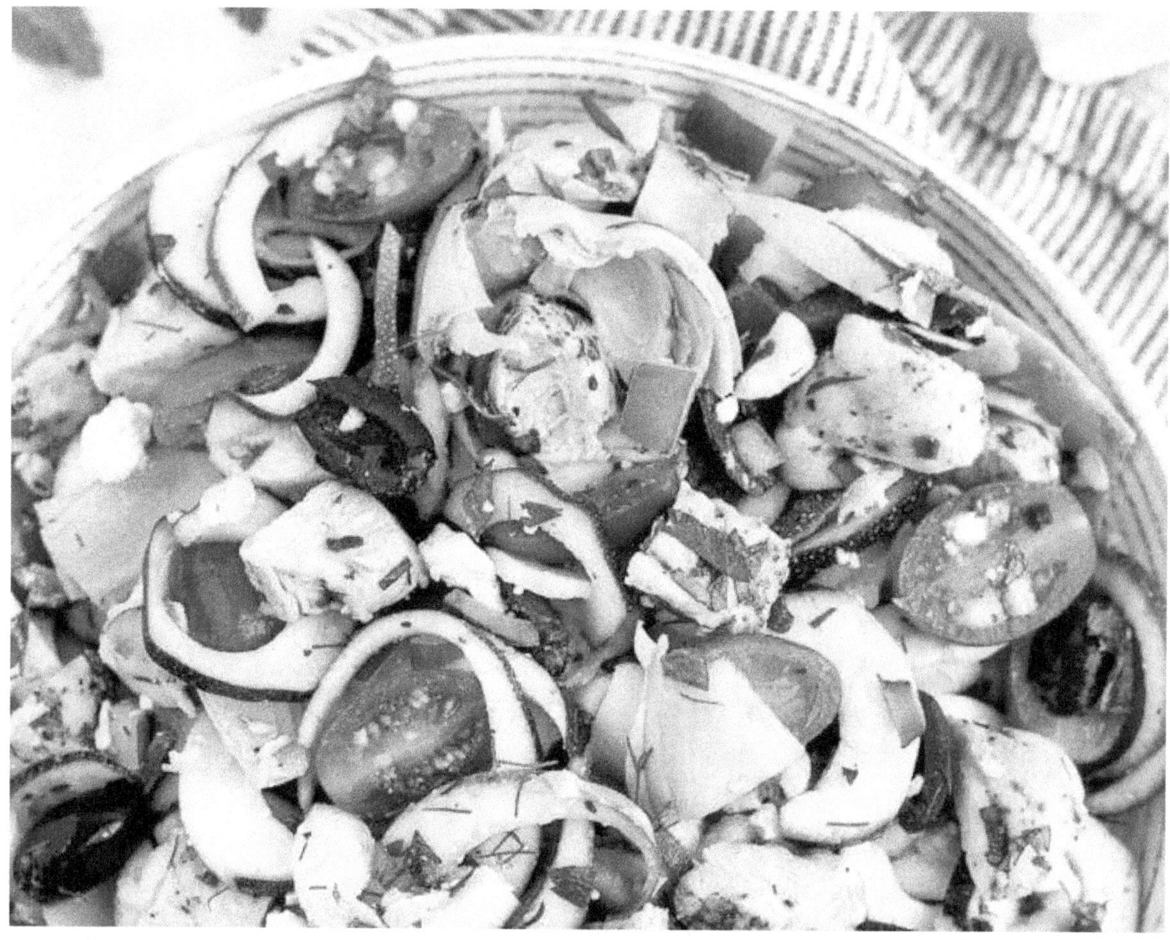

Whether served as main meal or as a side dish, this zucchini salad is sure to impress. But that's not all. It's also light and healthy.

Serving Size: 6

Preparation Cooking Time: 2 hours

Ingredients:

- 6 tablespoons olive oil, divided
- 2 chicken breast fillets
- Salt and pepper to taste
- 4 zucchinis, sliced into thin strips
- 15 oz. chickpeas, rinsed and drained
- 6 oz. black olives, pitted and sliced
- 14 oz. artichoke hearts, trimmed and chopped
- ½ cup Parmesan cheese, grated

Instructions:

1. First, sprinkle both sides of the chicken breast with the salt and pepper.

2. Pour 2 tablespoons olive oil into a pan over medium heat.

3. Cook the chicken breast for 5 to 8 minutes per side.

4. Slice the chicken into cubes.

5. Place in a bowl.

6. Next, pour the remaining oil in the same pan.

7. Cook the zucchini for 5 minutes.

8. Season with the salt and pepper.

9. Drain the zucchini on a plate lined with paper towel.

10. Combine the chickpeas, artichoke hearts and olives in a bowl.

11. Stir in the zucchini and sprinkle with the Parmesan cheese.

12. Refrigerate for 1 hour.

Nutrients per Serving:

- *Calories 75*
- *Fat 5 g*
- *Saturated fat 1 g*
- *Carbohydrates 26 g*
- *Fiber 5 g*
- *Protein 32 g*
- *Cholesterol 12 mg*
- *Sugars 2 g*
- *Sodium* 351 mg
- *Potassium 449 mg*

Grape Broccoli Salad

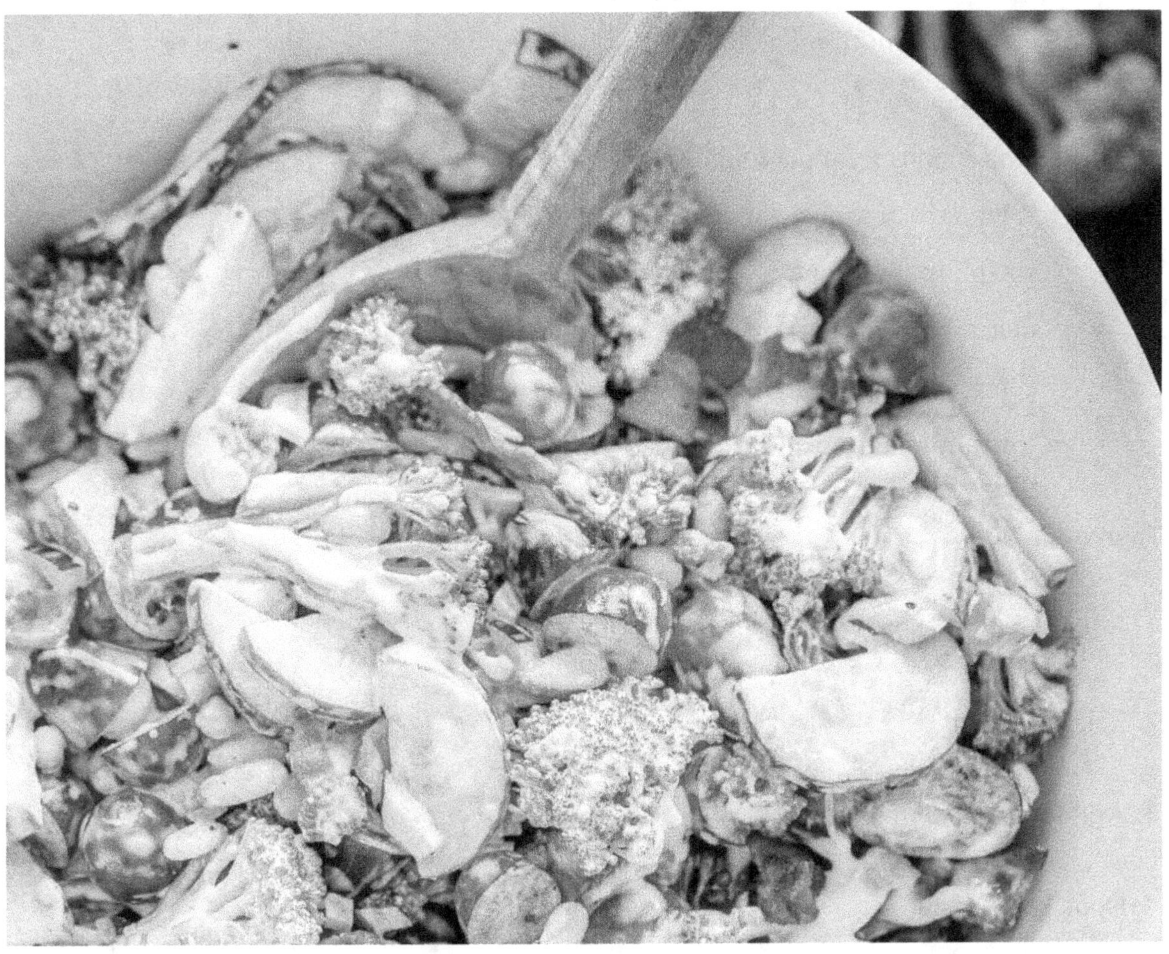

Grapes and broccoli—most people don't put this together in one dish. But this salad recipe would surprise you. You'll probably tell yourself that you should have discovered this incredible pairing sooner.

Serving Size: 4

Preparation Cooking Time: 20 minutes

Ingredients:

- ½ cup onion, chopped
- 3 cups broccoli florets
- ¼ cup reduced-fat Greek yogurt
- 3 tablespoons light mayonnaise
- 1 ½ tablespoons cider vinegar
- 1 ½ tablespoons honey
- Salt and pepper to taste
- 1 cup grapes, sliced in half
- ¼ cup almonds, toasted and sliced

Instructions:

1. Fill a pot with water.

2. Bring to a boil.

3. Add the onion and broccoli.

4. Cook for 2 minutes.

5. Drain and rinse the veggies in cold water.

6. Chill in the refrigerator.

7. In a bowl, combine the mayonnaise, yogurt, honey and vinegar.

8. Season with the salt and pepper.

9. Toss the broccoli and onions with the almonds and grapes.

10. Stir in the sauce.

11. Coat evenly.

Nutrients per Serving:

- *Calories 196*
- *Fat 11.7 g*
- *Saturated fat 1.9 g*
- *Carbohydrates 20.4 g*
- *Fiber 2.9 g*
- *Protein 5.1 g*
- *Cholesterol 6 mg*
- *Sugars 15 g*
- *Sodium 381 mg*
- *Potassium 380 mg*

Asparagus Soup

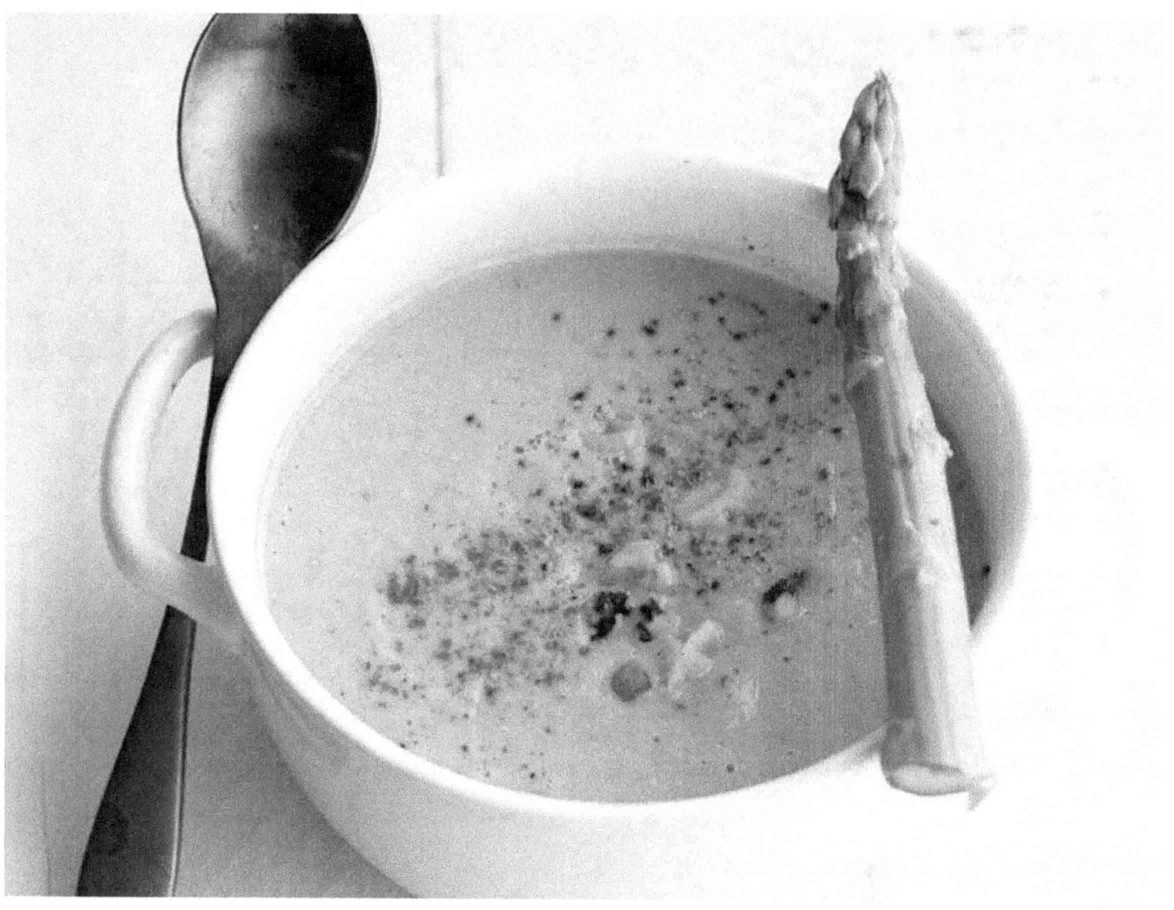

Prepare this comforting soup when you're craving for something tasty and creamy. It's made with asparagus, dill, spinach and roasted salmon, and topped with croutons, cucumber and sour cream.

Serving Size: 5

Preparation Cooking Time: 40 minutes

Ingredients:

- 12 oz. salmon fillet
- Cooking spray
- 1 lb. asparagus, trimmed and sliced
- ½ cup onion, chopped
- 1 tablespoon vegetable oil
- 29 oz. canned chicken broth
- 2 ½ cups nonfat milk
- ½ cup flour
- Salt to taste
- 1 tablespoon fresh dillweed, snipped
- 2 cups fresh spinach, chopped
- 5 tablespoons sour cream
- 1 slice rye bread, toasted and sliced into cubes
- ¼ cup cucumber, chopped

Instructions:

1. Preheat your oven to 450 degrees F.

2. Cover your baking pan with foil.

3. Spray the foil with oil.

4. Add the salmon on one side of the pan.

5. Place the asparagus on the other side.

6. Spray with the oil.

7. Roast in the oven for 5 minutes.

8. Flake the salmon.

9. Next, in your pan over medium heat, add the oil and cook for 5 minutes.

10. Pour in the broth.

11. In a bowl, mix the flour, salt and milk.

12. Pour into the pan.

13. Cook for 1 minute, stirring.

14. Stir in the salmon flakes, asparagus and dillweed.

15. Cook for 2 minutes.

16. Then, add the spinach and cook for 1 more minute.

17. Serve in soup bowls, topped with the rye croutons, sour cream and cucumber.

Nutrients per Serving:

- *Calories 318*
- *Fat 13.7 g*
- *Saturated fat 3.2 g*
- *Carbohydrates 24.9 g*
- *Fiber 2.4 g*
- *Protein 24 g*
- *Cholesterol 44 mg*
- *Sugars 9 g*
- *Sodium 603 mg*
- *Potassium 695 mg*

Frittata

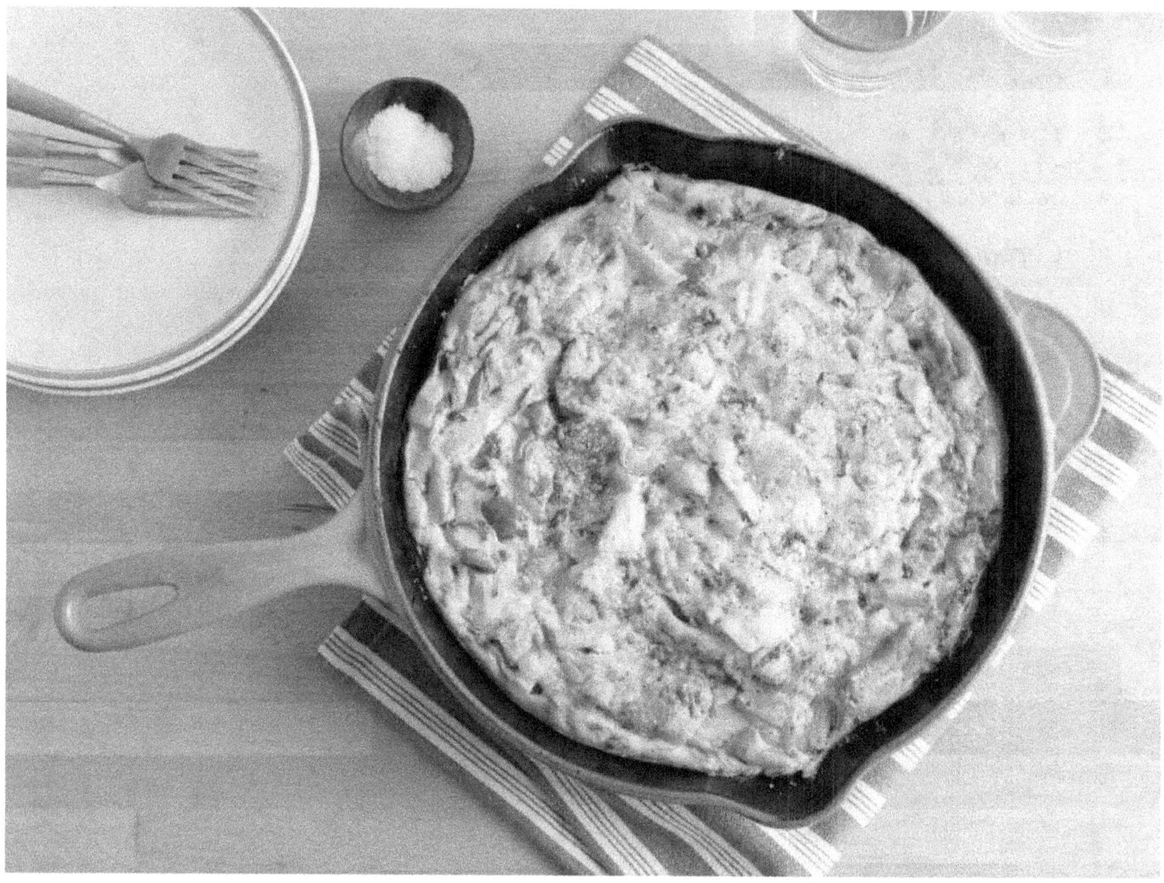

There are many ways to make frittata. It is one of the most delicious and easiest ways to make it. It's also colorful and vibrant as well.

Serving Size: 8

Preparation Cooking Time: 9 hours and 30 minutes

Ingredients:

- 1 lb. ground turkey breast
- 1 teaspoon onion powder
- ¼ teaspoon ground nutmeg
- ½ teaspoon dried sage, crushed
- 1/8 teaspoon dried marjoram
- ¼ teaspoon red pepper flakes
- Pepper to taste
- 3 whole-wheat muffins
- 4 eggs
- 2 cups nonfat milk
- ¼ teaspoon paprika
- 1 teaspoon dry mustard
- ¼ cup scallions, chopped
- 2 red peppers, chopped
- 2 green peppers, chopped
- 4 oz. low-fat cheddar cheese, shredded

Instructions:

1. In a bowl, mix the ground turkey, onion powder, nutmeg, sage, marjoram, red pepper flakes and pepper.

2. Transfer the mixture to a pan over medium heat.

3. Cook until brown.

4. Spray your baking pan with oil.

5. Slice the muffins and arrange in a single layer in the baking pan.

6. Sprinkle the turkey mixture on top.

7. In another bowl, beat the milk and eggs.

8. Season with the paprika, mustard and salt.

9. Pour the mixture on top.

10. Sprinkle the scallions and bell peppers on top.

11. Preheat your oven to 350 degrees F.

12. Bake for 45 minutes.

13. Top with the cheese.

14. Bake for another 5 minutes.

Nutrients per Serving:

- *Calories 235*
- *Fat 6.4 g*
- *Saturated fat 2.6 g*
- *Carbohydrates 16.7 g*
- *Fiber 2.6 g*
- *Protein 27.8 g*
- *Cholesterol 142 mg*
- *Sugars 7 g*
- *Sodium 448 mg*
- *Potassium 325 mg*

Cauliflower Rice Bowls

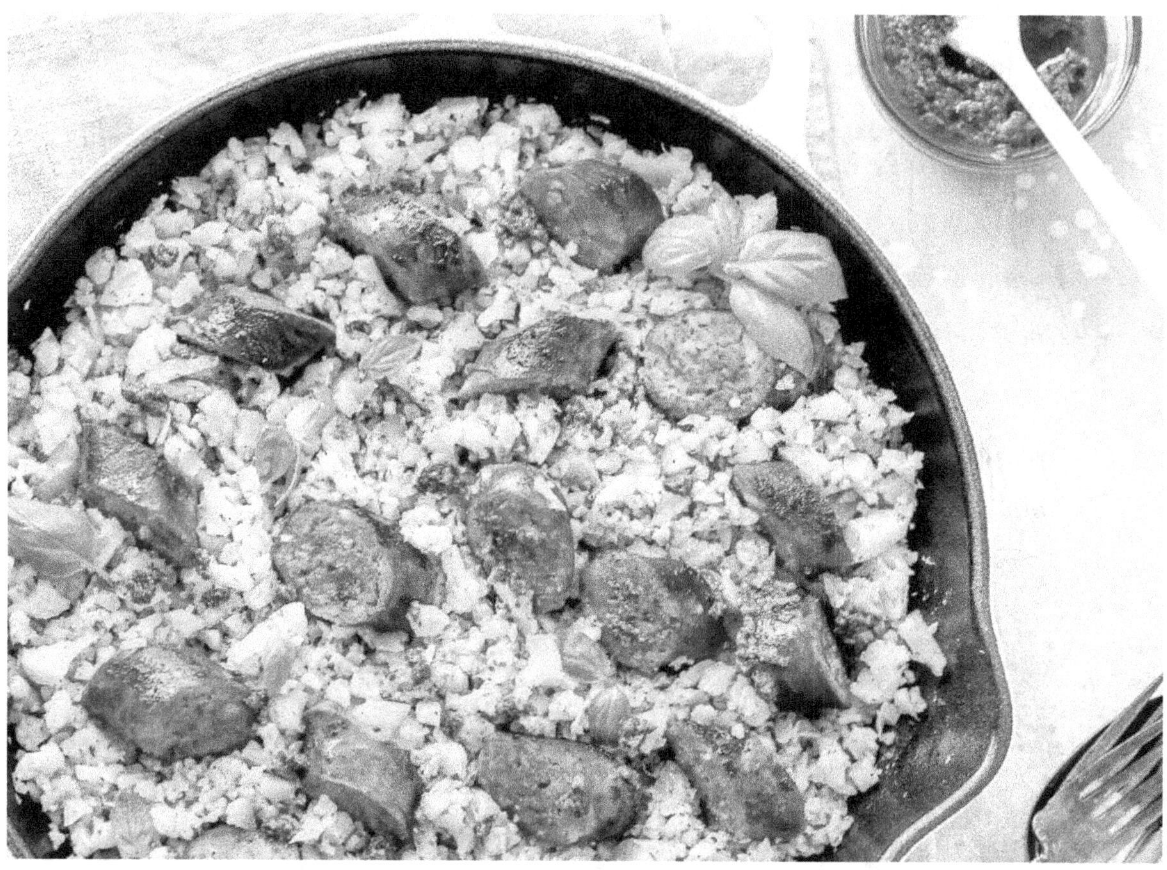

Cauliflower rice is not only for those who are on a low-carb diet, but anyone who wishes to eat healthier. Top it with nutritious fruits and veggies like avocado, asparagus and so on.

Serving Size: 4

Preparation Cooking Time: 15 minutes

Ingredients:

- 2 teaspoons olive oil
- 4 links Italian sausage, sliced
- 12 oz. asparagus spears
- 12 oz. cauliflower rice
- 6 tablespoons pesto

Instructions:

1. Pour the oil into a pan over medium heat.

2. Cook the sausage for 5 minutes per side.

3. Microwave the asparagus and cauliflower rice for 4 minutes.

4. Let cool.

5. Assemble the rice bowls by topping the rice with the asparagus and sausage and serving it with pesto.

Nutrients per Serving:

- *Calories 290*
- *Fat 19.4 g*
- *Saturated fat 4.1 g*
- *Carbohydrates 7.5 g*
- *Fiber 3.5 g*
- *Protein 20.4 g*
- *Cholesterol 65 mg*
- *Sugars 2 g*
- *Sodium 733 mg*
- *Potassium 193 mg*

Kale Soup

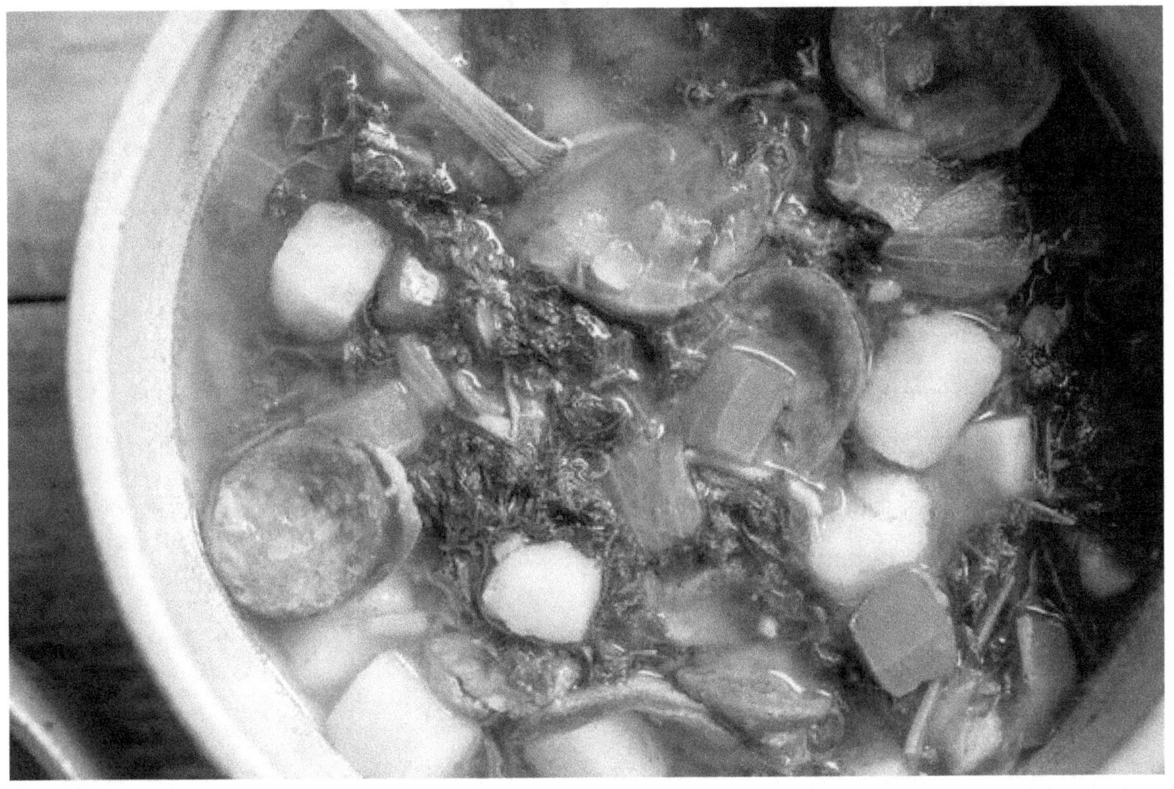

This kale soup gives you comfort with every sip. It's made with beans, spinach and potatoes.

Serving Size: 8

Preparation Cooking Time: 1 hour

Ingredients:

- 1 onion, chopped
- 2 tablespoons olive oil
- 8 cups water
- 6 cubes vegetable bouillon
- 1 kale, chopped
- 2 tablespoons garlic, chopped
- 15 oz. canned diced tomatoes
- 6 potatoes, sliced into cubes
- 2 tablespoons dried 30 oz. cannellini beans
- parsley
- 1 tablespoon Italian seasoning
- Salt and pepper to taste

Instructions:

1. Pour the olive oil into a pot over medium heat.

2. Cook the onion for 1 minute.

3. Next, add the garlic. Cook for 30 seconds.

4. Then, add the kale. Cook while stirring for 2 minutes.

5. Add the rest of the ingredients.

6. Reduce heat and simmer for 25 minutes.

Nutrients per Serving:

- *Calories 277*
- *Fat 4.5 g*
- *Saturated fat 1 g*
- *Carbohydrates 50.9 g*
- *Fiber 10.3 g*
- *Protein 9.6 g*
- *Cholesterol 0 mg*
- *Sugars 5 g*
- *Sodium 372 mg*
- *Potassium 1042 mg*

Black Beans in a Bowl

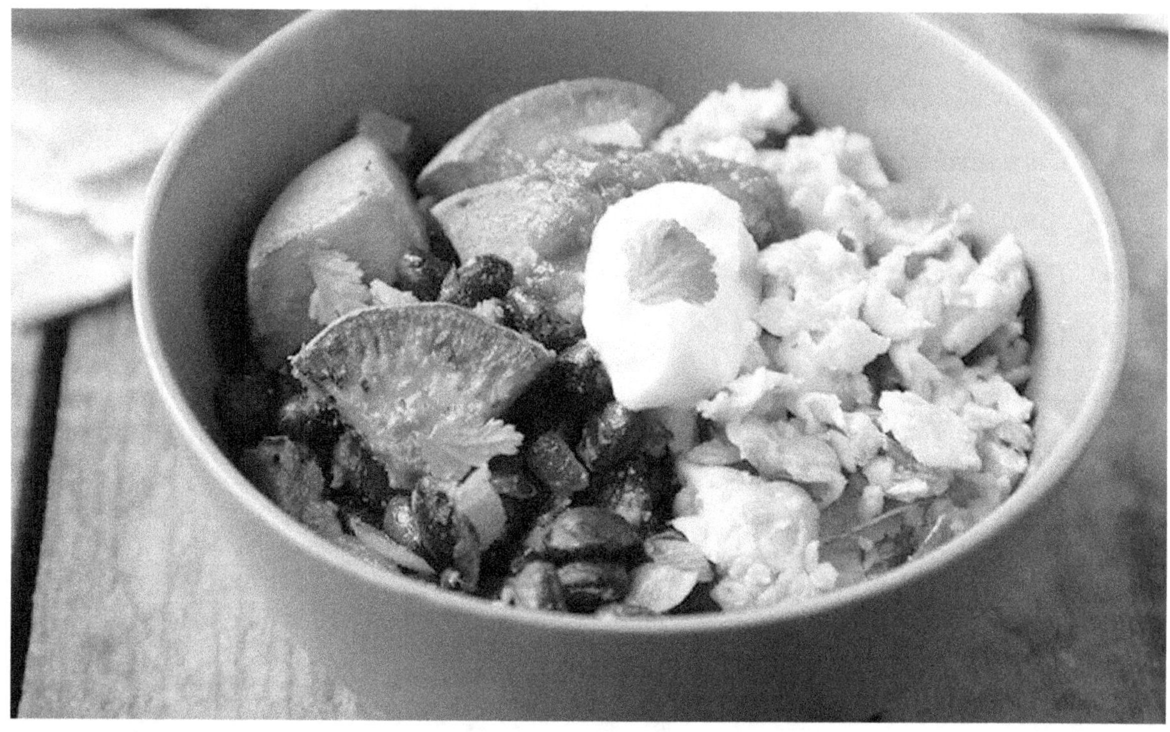

Here's how you can enjoy black beans even more—serve these with eggs, salsa and avocado.

Serving Size: 2

Preparation Cooking Time: 15 minutes

Ingredients:

- 2 tablespoons olive oil
- 1 avocado, peeled and sliced
- 4 eggs, beaten
- 15 oz. canned black bean, rinsed and drained
- ¼ cup salsa
- Salt and pepper to taste

Instructions:

1. Pour the olive oil into a pan over medium heat.

2. Cook the eggs for 4 to 5 minutes.

3. Add the black beans in a heat-proof bowl.

4. Microwave on high for 1 minute.

5. Add the eggs, black beans and the rest of the ingredients in serving bowls.

6. Season with the salt and pepper.

Nutrients per Serving:

- *Calories 625*
- *Fat 38.8 g*
- *Saturated fat 7 g*
- *Carbohydrates 46.6 g*
- *Fiber 21.9 g*
- *Protein 27.9 g*
- *Cholesterol 372 mg*
- *Sugars 2 g*
- *Sodium 1158 mg*
- *Potassium 1372 mg*

Grilled Fish with Tomatoes Spinach

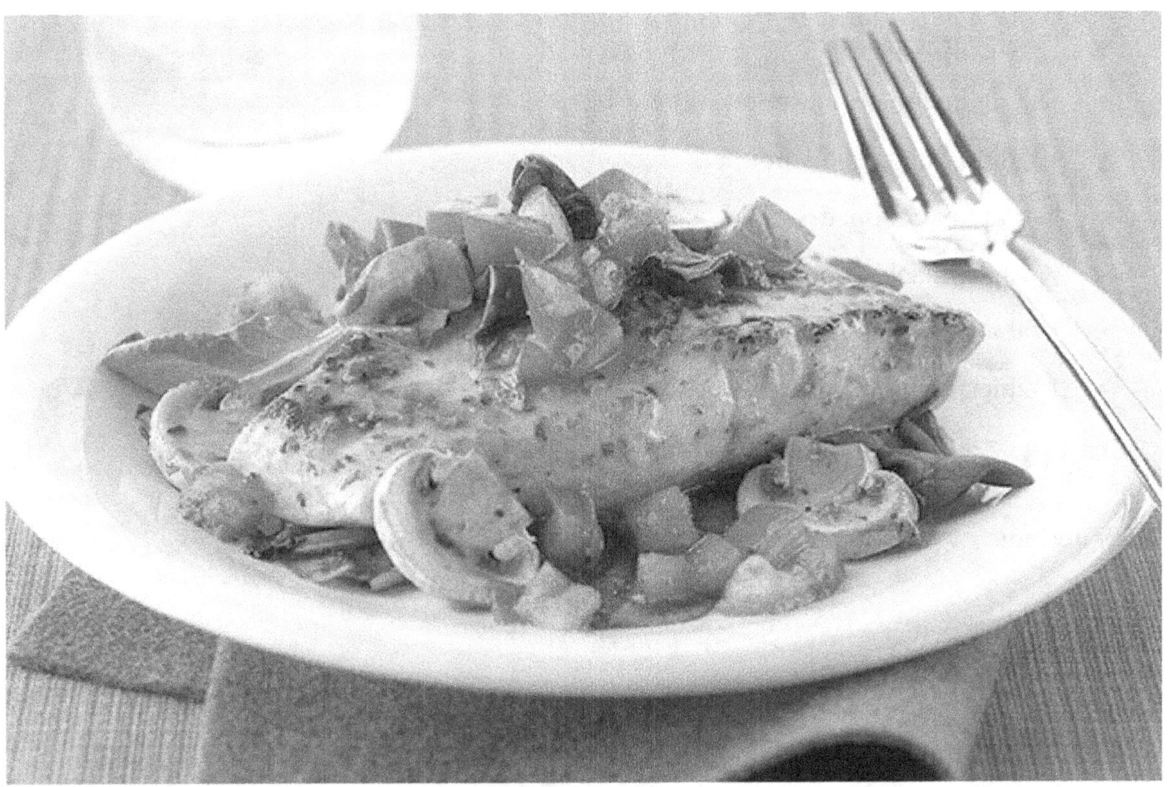

Running out of ideas come dinner time? Here's a simple and tasty meal—grilled fish with the spinach and cherry tomatoes.

Serving Size: 1

Preparation Cooking Time: 20 minutes

Ingredients:

- 1 cod fillet
- Pinch garlic powder
- Salt and pepper to taste
- 1 tablespoon onion, chopped
- ¼ tomato, chopped
- ¼ cup spinach, chopped
- 1 tablespoon balsamic vinegar
- 1 tablespoon olive oil
- 1 mozzarella cheese slice, cut into smaller cubes

Instructions:

1. Preheat your grill.

2. Season the fish with the garlic powder, salt and pepper.

3. Place on a foil sheet.

4. Top the fish with the onion, tomato and spinach.

5. Drizzle the vinegar and olive on top.

6. Arrange the slices of mozzarella cheese on top of the fish.

7. Wrap the fish and veggies with foil.

8. Grill the packet for 10 minutes, flipping once.

Nutrients per Serving:

- *Calories 308*
- *Fat 18.9 g*
- *Saturated fat 5 g*
- *Carbohydrates 6.4 g*
- *Fiber 0.9 g*
- *Protein 27.8 g*
- *Cholesterol 66 mg*
- *Sugars 4 g*
- *Sodium 413 mg*
- *Potassium 419 mg*

Grilled Chicken with Fruits

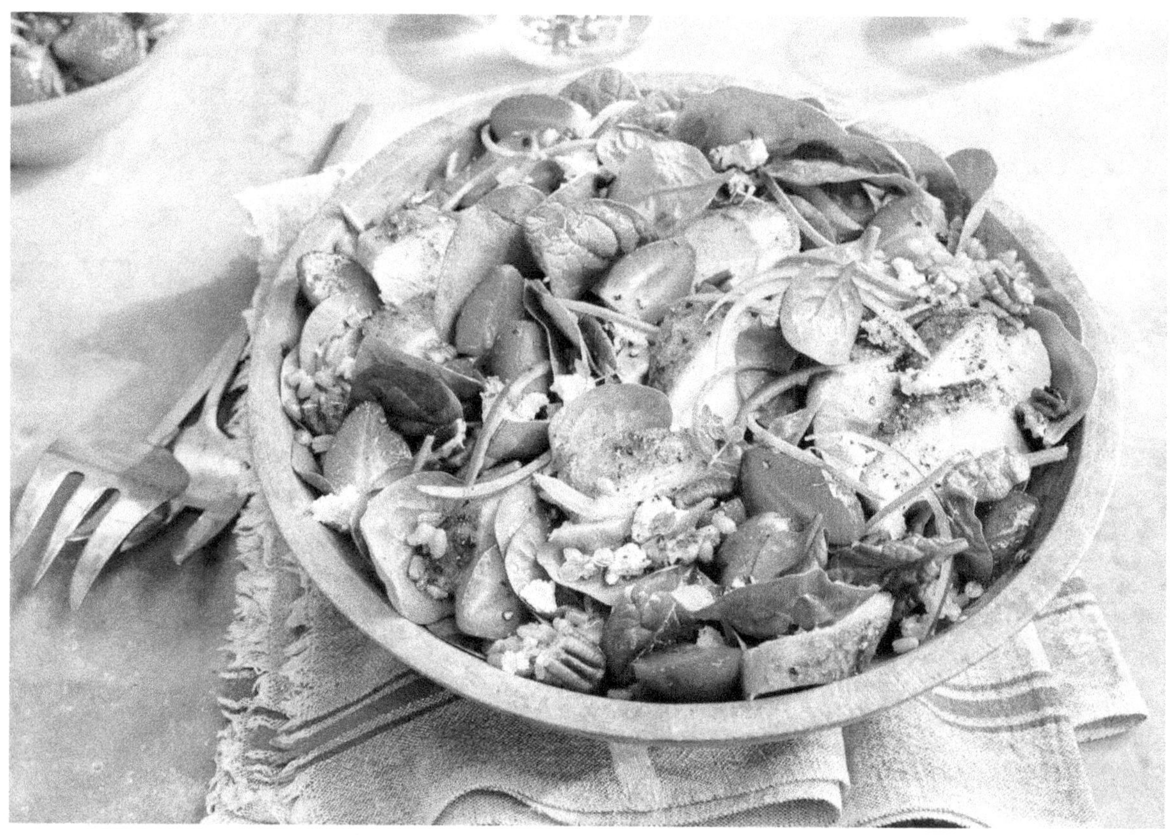

All Of the chicken salad recipes you've seen, this is probably the most colorful. It also won't disappoint your taste buds with its sweet and savory flavors.

Serving Size: 6

Preparation Cooking Time: 35 minutes

Ingredients:

- 1 lb. chicken breast fillet
- ½ cup pecans
- ¼ cup red wine vinegar
- ½ cup white sugar
- 1 cup vegetable oil
- ½ onion, minced
- 1 teaspoon ground mustard
- Salt and pepper to taste
- 2 heads lettuce, rinsed and chopped
- 1 cup fresh strawberries, sliced

Instructions:

1. Preheat your grill.

2. Grill the chicken for 8 minutes per side.

3. Remove from the grill and slice.

4. Add the pecans and toast in the pan.

5. Next, cook for 8 to 10 minutes, stirring frequently.

6. Add the rest of the ingredients in a blender.

7. Then, pulse until smooth.

8. Place the lettuce leaves on plates.

9. Top the lettuce leaves with the chicken, pecans and strawberries.

10. Pour the dressing on top and serve.

Nutrients per Serving:

- *Calories 567*
- *Fat 46 g*
- *Saturated fat 5.9 g*
- *Carbohydrates 23.2 g*
- *Fiber 2.3 g*
- *Protein 17.8 g*
- *Cholesterol 43 mg*
- *Sugars 19 g*
- *Sodium 428 mg*
- *Potassium 367 mg*

White Bean Soup

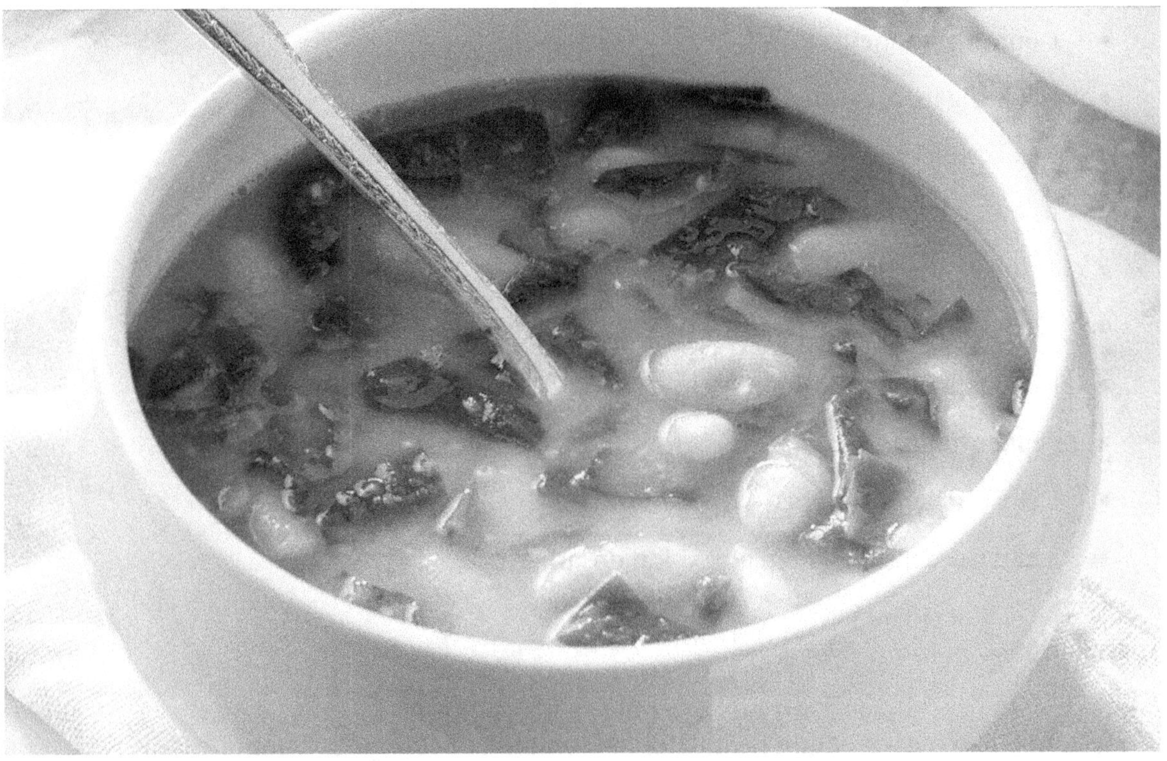

Make this healthy and delicious white bean soup without spending too much time in the kitchen.

Serving Size: 4

Preparation Cooking Time: 50 minutes

Ingredients:

- 1 tablespoon vegetable oil
- 1 onion, chopped
- 1 clove garlic, crushed and minced
- 1 stalk celery, chopped
- 14 oz. chicken broth
- 2 cups water
- 32 oz. white kidney beans, rinsed and drained
- 1/8 teaspoon dried thyme
- Pepper to taste
- 1 cup spinach, chopped
- 1 tablespoon freshly squeezed lemon juice

Instructions:

1. First, in a pan over medium heat, cook the onion and celery for 5 minutes.

2. Add the garlic and cook until fragrant.

3. Stir in the chicken broth, water, kidney beans, thyme and pepper.

4. Bring to a boil.

5. Reduce heat and simmer for 15 minutes.

6. Next, transfer 2 cups of the bean mixture to a bowl.

7. Add the remaining mixture to a blender.

8. Pulse until smooth.

9. Put the mixture back to the pot.

10. Add the reserved beans into the pot.

11. Bring to a boil.

12. Add the spinach.

13. Cook for 1 minute.

14. Add the lemon juice.

15. Serve warm.

Nutrients per Serving:

- *Calories 245*
- *Fat 4.9 g*
- *Saturated fat 1 g*
- *Carbohydrates 38.1 g*
- *Fiber 11.2 g*
- *Protein 12 g*
- *Cholesterol 2 mg*
- *Sugars 2 g*
- *Sodium 1014 mg*
- *Potassium 551 mg*

Conclusion

Not only will you have enjoyable creating these awesome dishes, you'll also be delighted with the immediate benefits you'll get.

You'll experience fewer or milder episodes of morning sickness, feel better and less tired, and have more energy to do what you need to do prepare for your baby's arrival.

Plus, these recipes are also easy enough that even if you are in your third trimester, you won't find any of these too challenging.

As you are perfectly aware of, being pregnant is not easy. But it's even more difficult when your baby is already here.

Good nutrition is a good investment to make. It will not only help you with labor and delivery but will also help ensure the health and safety of your little one.

And of course, that's what matters most.

Use this cookbook to start your pregnancy journey with healthy diet.

About the Author

A native of Albuquerque, New Mexico, Sophia Freeman found her calling in the culinary arts when she enrolled at the Sante Fe School of Cooking. Freeman decided to take a year after graduation and travel around Europe, sampling the cuisine from small bistros and family owned restaurants from Italy to Portugal. Her bubbly personality and inquisitive nature made her popular with the locals in the villages and when she finished her trip and came home, she had made friends for life in the places she had visited. She also came home with a deeper understanding of European cuisine.

Freeman went to work at one of Albuquerque's 5-star restaurants as a sous-chef and soon worked her way up to head chef. The restaurant began to feature Freeman's original dishes as specials on the menu and soon after, she began to write e-books with her recipes. Sophia's dishes mix local flavours with European inspiration making them irresistible to the diners in her restaurant and the online community.

Freeman's experience in Europe didn't just teach her new ways of cooking, but also unique methods of presentation. Using rich sauces, crisp vegetables and meat cooked to perfection, she creates a stunning display as well as a delectable dish. She has won many local awards for her cuisine and she continues to delight her diners with her culinary masterpieces.

Author's Afterthoughts

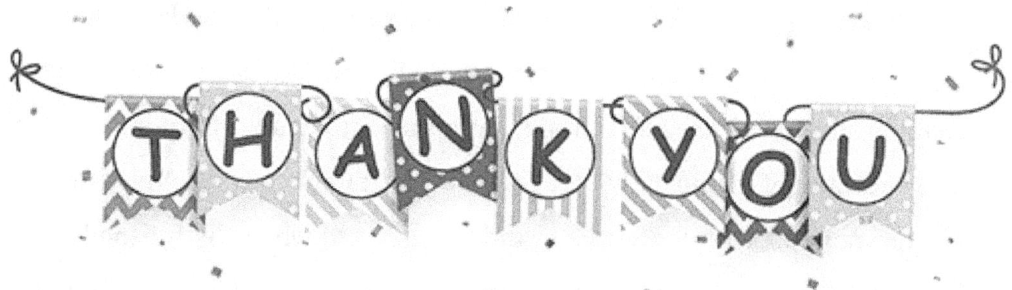

I want to convey my big thanks to all of my readers who have taken the time to read my book. Readers like you make my work so rewarding and I cherish each and every one of you.

Grateful cannot describe how I feel when I know that someone has chosen my work over all of the choices available online. I hope you enjoyed the book as much as I enjoyed writing it.

Feedback from my readers is how I grow and learn as a chef and an author. Please take the time to let me know your thoughts by leaving a review on Amazon so I and your fellow readers can learn from your experience.

My deepest thanks,

Sophia Freeman

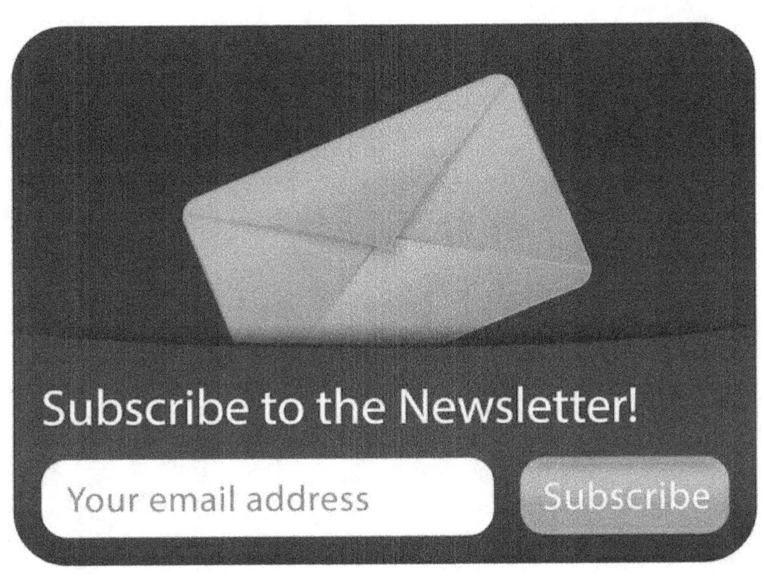

https://sophia.subscribemenow.com/

* * * * ★ ★ ★ ★ ★ * * *

www.ingramcontent.com/pod-product-compliance
Lightning Source LLC
Chambersburg PA
CBHW081304250726
48662CB00008B/2390